Dr. Ellington Darden's
SECRET
to Reclaim Your Youth

By Don Brown
Fitness Entrepreneur

People between 45 and 70 years of age in the United States need more muscle and less fat and Ellington Darden's decades of research provides transforming help for aging bodies. That's why I'm pleased to write the foreword for his latest book, *Still Living Longer Stronger*.

Our journey began 40 years ago when we first crossed paths in 1983 at a Nautilus Fitness Seminar in DeLand, Florida. At that time, you were the Director of Research for Nautilus, introducing an innovative idea: *Negative* Strength Training. "It's not about how much weight you can lift," you said, "it's about how much weight you can lower slowly." This simple yet revolutionary practice laid the foundation for your extensive work in strength training and fat loss.

Over these decades, we've become more than just friends. We've been partners in the world of fitness, and I've had the privilege of introducing some of my inventions into the mix. As a fitness entrepreneur and inventor, I've witnessed the impact of your groundbreaking concepts on countless individuals. It was great for me to work alongside you when I launched the AB Trainer infomercial in 1993, an experience that further solidified our shared commitment to empowering people with the knowledge and tools to improve their lives.

Since then, you've authored an astounding 40 books on various techniques to increase muscle mass while shedding body fat. I eagerly purchased each one, applying the principles to my own training and the members of my health club in New Jersey. Your books became the programs I offered to my community, courses like *Two Weeks to a Tighter Tummy*, *32 Days to a 32-Inch Waist*, *Hot Hips and Fabulous Thighs*, and many more. Thousands of my health club members have reaped the benefits of your wisdom.

I opened my first health club at the age of 27, and today, at 65, I can confidently say that I am living stronger than I ever thought possible. I can still do 17 pull-ups, run a 7-minute mile, and perform 40 push-ups in one minute. Plus, my mobility remains at a high level. All my exercise success is a direct result of your unwavering dedication to research in the field of strength training.

And this brings us to why I am writing the foreword for your book. *Still Living Longer Stronger* contains the most significant secret known to both men and women for adding years to their lives. The concept is a major advance for rebuilding youthful muscle, potentially slowing, or even reversing the effects of aging. This secret is your "10-10-10 Method," and it only requires a 15-minute routine, twice a week.

When used, this secret won't merely add years to your life, it may prevent you from ever needing a walker, cane, or wheelchair. So, if you are interested in making your 70s, 80s, and 90s as good as your 50s and 60s, then start reading and focusing.

It's time to apply Dr. Darden's secret and reclaim your youth.

10-10-10

Still Living Longer Stronger

Best Selling Books
by Ellington Darden, PhD

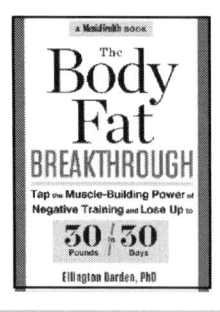

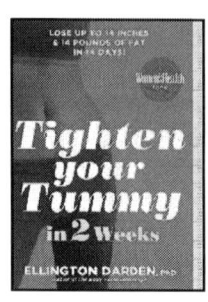

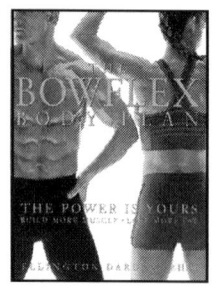

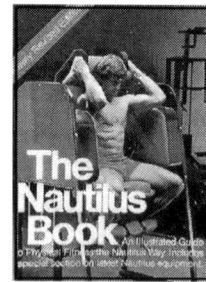

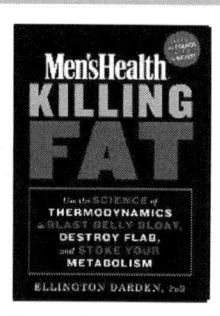

Over 21 Best Selling Books

written by Ellington Darden helping both
men and women live leaner and stronger lives!

- Strength-Training Principles • Conditioning for Football
- The Athlete's Guide to Sports Medicine
- The Complete Encyclopedia of Weight Loss,
  Body Shaping, and Slenderizing
- The Nautilus Book • The Nautilus Bodybuilding Book
- The Nautilus Diet • The Six-Week Fat-to-Muscle Makeover
- High-Intensity Bodybuilding • Super High-Intensity Bodybuilding
- 32 Days to a 32-Inch Waist • Hot Hips and Fabulous Thighs
- Bigger Muscles in 42 Days • Soft Steps to a Hard Body
- A Flat Stomach ASAP • The Bowflex Body Plan
- The New High Intensity Training • The Body Fat Breakthrough
- The New Bodybuilding for Old-School Results
- Flat Belly Breakthrough for Women • Men's Health Killing Fat

available at
amazon

Still Living Longer Stronger

- Feel 20 years younger in just 6 weeks.
- Extend and enhance your years over 50.
- Reduce, rebuild, and rejuvenate . . . NOW!

Ellington Darden, PhD
World Renowned Strength Training Expert

This book is intended as a reference guide only, not as a medical manual. The information given here is designed to help you make informed decisions about your health. It is not intended as a substitute for any treatment that may have been prescribed by your doctor. If you suspect that you have a medical problem, we urge you to seek competent medical help.

The information in this book is meant to supplement, not replace, proper exercise training. All forms of exercise pose some inherent risks. The editors and publisher advise readers to take full responsibility for their safety and know their limits. Before practicing the exercises in this book, be sure that your equipment is well-maintained, and do not take risks beyond your level of experience, aptitude, training, and fitness. The exercise and dietary programs in this book are not intended as a substitute for any exercise routine or dietary regimen that may have been prescribed by your doctor. As with all exercise and dietary programs, you should get your doctor's approval before beginning.

© 2024 by Ellington Darden, PhD

Library of Congress Cataloging-in-Publication Data: 2023917794

All rights reserved. No part of this publication may be reproduced or transmitted in any form or by any means, electronic or mechanical, including photocopying, recording, or any other information storage and retrieval system, without the written permission of the author.

Cover photograph by Jeanenne Darden.
Cover design by Greg Perri.
Before-and-after photographs © by Ellington Darden.
Illustration on page 31 by Karen Kuchar.
Casual photographs of women by Paul Privette.
Editing by Chisom Ezeh.

Special thanks to Don Brown for his inspiring concepts and overall support.

Distributed by The Publishing Pad
www.thepublishingpad.com

ISBN: 979-8-9880488-6-2 (Paperback)
ISBN: 979-8-9880488-7-9 (Hardcover)

Printed in the United States of America

Contents

A Tale of Two Covers 7

I Resolving Age-Old Problems 9
1. Moving Forward 10
2. See, Believe, Achieve 14
3. Biomarkers and Muscle 20
4. Disuse Atrophy and Creeping Obesity 26
5. Building Muscle and Losing Fat . . . Simultaneously 30
6. Not Just Stronger, But Enduring and Flexible 38

II Reexamining Strength Training and Nutrition 46
7. Negative Awakening, 10-10-10, and Lift & Lower-Slower ... 47
8. List of the Best 10-10-10 Exercises 59
9. Single-Joint Exercises 61
10. Multiple-Joint Exercises 76
11. Proactive Eating 89
12. Nutrition Fallacies and Facts 97

III Removing Excess Body Fat 105
13. Patterns of Fat Distribution 106
14. Losing Fat Through Your Skin 109
15. Watering Your Fat Away 114
16. Eat a Meal, Walk a Mile 123
17. The Importance of Extra Sleep 127
18. Hot News About Cold 133

IV Rebuilding and Reducing Programs 141
19. A 28-Pound Fat/Muscle Makeover 142
20. Before Getting Started 144
21. Overview of the SLLS Eating Program 153
22. The SLLS Eating Plan for Weeks 1-6 158
23. Living-Longer-Stronger Workouts For Weeks 1–6 166
24. Troubleshooting Guide 170
    Bonus Challenge! Can You Spare a Couple of Weeks? 180

V Rejuvenating Your Life 186
25 Improving Your Results.. 187
26 Maintenance Guidelines... 192
27 Advanced Strength Training Techniques and Workouts..... 196
28 "I Feel Twenty Years Younger!" 200
29 Dancing on Your Troubles.. 203
30 It's Still Working 207

VI Retelling Lost Stories: Memoirs 219
31 Mirror Shine... 222
32 Do You Have Change for a Dollar?................................. 231
33 Wanted: Dead or Alive!... 238
34 Good Vibrations.. 243
35 The Rest of Your Life 254
36 The Transition of Knowledge.. 261

Bibliography 272
7 Keys for Success 279

Free Gift
Still Living Longer Stronger 6 Week Program (free PDF) 280

A Tale of Two Covers

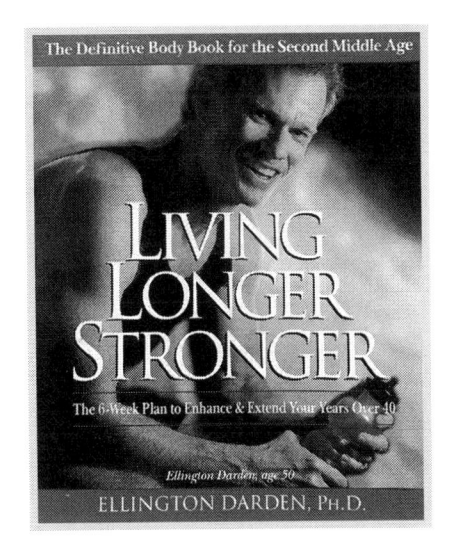

A 1995 review of my book *Living Longer Stronger* noted that the cover photo of me, with the light streaming through the darkness, must have been taken in Notre Dame's archaic, dimly lit weight room during the 1960s.

Years ago, *Strength & Health* magazine published pictures of Notre Dame's weight room, which was managed by Father Bernard Lange. As a longtime reader of the magazine, I remember those photos well. One of them showed sunlight flooding through an overhead window and across an athlete doing a standing barbell press.

Indeed, the photo of me on the cover of *Living Longer Stronger* did resemble that photo from *Strength & Health*. But the old-school feel was in fact created by Gene Bednarek of Gainesville, Florida, in his photography studio. Gene had high-quality cameras, lights, and background materials. Plus, Gene had a technique of slightly jarring the camera as the shutter closed, which produced a curious glow around the subject. The photoshoot lasted four hours—it took us that long to get the look we wanted.

Fast-forward to 2023. The picture of me on the cover of *Still Living Longer Stronger*—the book you are reading now—was taken by my wife, Jeanenne, with her iPhone 14. She asked me to assume a pose similar to the one on the old cover, right down to the water bottle in my hand, but she wanted a more modern look to the picture. The setting is my home office, with black closet doors in the background and no special lighting other than sunlight from the nearby windows. Jeanenne logged thirty-five shots of me in twenty minutes, and the best one is on the 2023 cover.

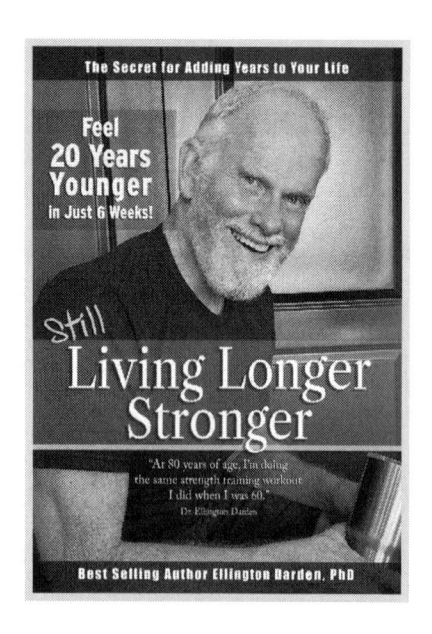

Photography, design, and layout used to require a lot of time. Every stage—from choosing the right film and setting up lights to chemical processing, color balancing, cropping, and printing—took a lot of doing and redoing. Today, all those components have been digitized, computerized, and sped up. Some would argue that the final product has not improved in proportion to the time saved. Others would disagree.

From 1995 to 2023 is twenty-eight years, and that's a long time. As Charles Dickens—the famous British novelist—might say, "It was the best of times, it was the worst of times. It was the age of wisdom, it was the age of madness."

A reporter once asked Arthur Jones, the man who invented Nautilus exercise machines, how old he was. His reply: "Old enough to know you can't change the thinking of fools, but young and foolish enough to keep on trying."

Two covers, two books—united. With stories worth telling and retelling.

A new you, boosted, updated, and revitalized. Age 80 is the new 60.

Get ready to change your life.

> All aboard for . . .
> **Still** Living Longer Stronger

I

RESOLVING AGE-OLD PROBLEMS

1

Still Living Longer Stronger

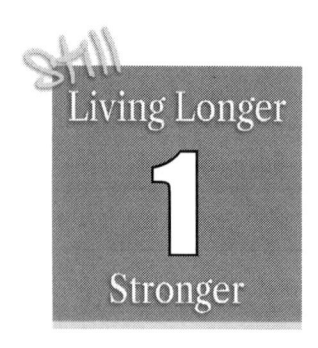

Moving Forward

A telephone conversation, February 23, 2023:

"**Still**," Don Brown said to me. "Just add that one word to the title of your 1995 book, *Living Longer Stronger*."

Don is the creator of such best-selling fitness products as AB Trainer, Ab Roller, and Stealth Core Trainer. More than thirty-five years ago, he also owned and operated a Nautilus Fitness Center in New Jersey, where I first met him.

"You may be right," I replied to Don. I had been searching for a book idea.

Don continued: "Fill your Living Longer Stronger followers in on what you've learned over the last three decades about strength training."

"Yes, there's been a lot of new research on muscle building and fat loss," I noted, "and I've applied it to my own body. The improved techniques are adaptable for almost anyone over 60 years of age."

"*Still Living Longer Stronger*," Don said, "is a great title, and it describes your book perfectly for the people who need it most."

Now Revised and Revitalized

My 1995 Living Longer Stronger program has been used successfully by more than 100,000 people. This 2023 version is not just reworked; it's supercharged, packed with the latest scientific techniques and breakthroughs so you can achieve success faster than ever.

The new program works for both men and women. In fact, many women over age 60 have neglected their muscles for most of their lives. As a result, they need to add muscle as much as men do—perhaps even more.

A revitalized, stronger body will allow you to live a healthier and more productive second middle age and beyond.

The Second Middle Age

In 1900, scientists divided a person's life into three stages: youth, defined as birth to age 20; middle age, from age 21 to 40; and old age, from age 41 to death. The average person living in the United States at the beginning of the twentieth century could expect to die at age 47. The prevalent belief then was that people over 40 could not be creative or productive.

More than 120 years later, life expectancy for Americans is 80 years—and gradually increasing with each new set of statistics that's released. As a result, there's an emerging "second middle age" that we need to take advantage of.

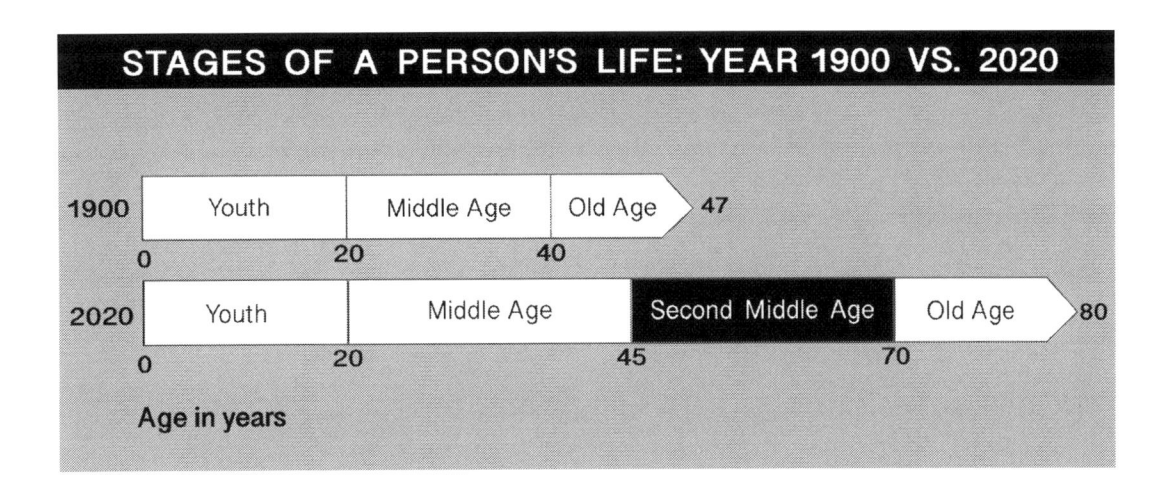

STAGES OF A PERSON'S LIFE: YEAR 1900 VS. 2020

Year					
1900	Youth (0–20)	Middle Age (20–40)	Old Age (40–47)		
2020	Youth (0–20)	Middle Age (20–45)	Second Middle Age (45–70)	Old Age (70–80)	

Age in years

The concept of a second middle age was introduced by Dr. Lydia Bronte in her 1993 book *The Longevity Factor*. In 1995, I narrowed her concept to men only and defined the second middle age as a stage of manhood between the ages of 40 and 60. Since then, however, I have included women in the mix.

I have also expanded my definition of the second middle age. Today, my first middle age goes from 21 to 45, and the second middle age extends from 46 to 70 years of age. Why the expansion? The answer is simple. People are living longer. An individual celebrating his or her 70th birthday should be preparing for another decade or two of creative adulthood. Tragically, many men and women remain ill-prepared for this journey.

The second middle age in a person's life can be an exciting, pivotal time. It's a time to look back, evaluate, learn, apply, and move forward. *Restore, retrain, rethink, relearn, rebuild,* and *renew* are the challenges of the fifth, sixth, seventh, and eighth decades of life.

Successfully dealing with the second middle age enables people to boldly enter their twilight years—those after age 70—armed with knowledge of healthy habits that are easy to stick with. Statistics reveal that most Americans die not simply from a particular disease, but from how they chose to live. This book is about distinguishing wise choices from foolish ones.

Yes, the last ten years of life (for example, from 70 to 80 or from 80 to 90) are frequently judged to be old age. But with this book, they can become some of your most self-assured and confident years.

A Muscular Foundation

The foundation of this book is the extensive research I've been doing since 1965. My studies prove that muscles are the engines of the body. They perform work. They demand energy. They produce movement. They offer protection.

Building stronger muscles is the single best medicine you can prescribe for yourself. Stronger muscles fend off degeneration. Stronger muscles escalate productivity. Stronger muscles are the key to living longer.

The oldest members of the post–World War II generation, the baby boomers, have reached their late 70s. Not only do some of them deny being over the hill, but many are broadening their horizons with different challenges.

The supercharged *Still Living Longer Stronger* is designed to help every baby boomer meet those challenges. Interestingly, most of these boomers want a strong core, and my program hits that area intensely.

For more than six decades, I've been actively involved in strength training and bodybuilding. "Bodybuilding" may bring to your mind images of oiled, shaved bodies in tiny trunks, posing and flexing their muscles. Yes, competitive body building does require a good bit of muscular display. But the type of bodybuilding and strength training in this course is about developing your muscles for performance, leanness, fitness, and health. I'm talking about muscles that display that inherent youthful vitality.

Step-By-Step Progress

In 1900, there were only 122,000 people in the United States age 85 or older. By 2030, it is projected that Americans age 85 and older will number 17.5 million. Very few societies in the history of humanity have ever had such an opportunity for continued productivity and adventure.

Each chapter in parts I through III of this book supplies easy-to-follow guidelines and inspiration on living a stronger, leaner, longer, and more fruitful life. Part IV incorporates those guidelines into an effective plan. Follow it for six weeks, and you'll reduce your body fat, flatten your stomach, reinforce your lower back, hydrate your systems, firm up your arms and chest, strengthen your legs, and improve your heart-lung endurance.

You and your friends will be amazed at your improved body and your new outlook.

My 10-10-10 method of strength training will rebuild and build your muscles to new levels. I can almost guarantee your best-possible results.

We're moving forward. *Still.*

Still Living Longer 2 Stronger

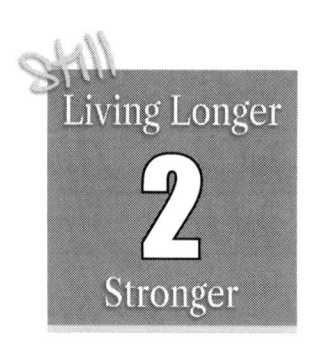

See, Believe, Achieve

The eyes rule the senses. What we see—more than what we hear, feel, taste, or smell—is what we tend to believe.

That's why I take before-and-after photographs (front, side, and back views) of all people who go through my programs. At the end of each course, I make prints and invite participants to a meeting to view and compare the results. Such viewings—I have done thousands of them—and the pride and enthusiasm they generate are the best advertising for recruiting and motivating people for the next program.

Participants in my research studies sign release forms that allow me to use their pictures, as well as their names, measurements, questionnaires, and interviews, in my publications. You might think that my subjects would want to guard their privacy. But once they see their amazing results, they can't wait to share what they've achieved—because they hope to inspire others, like you.

> "Ellington Darden's technical command of taking and using before-and-after photography sets him apart from his competition in fat-loss and muscle-building books. His books are not only scientifically sound and amazingly effective, they are believable and inspirational."
>
> **Joe Cirulli,**
> owner and manager of
> Gainesville Health & Fitness

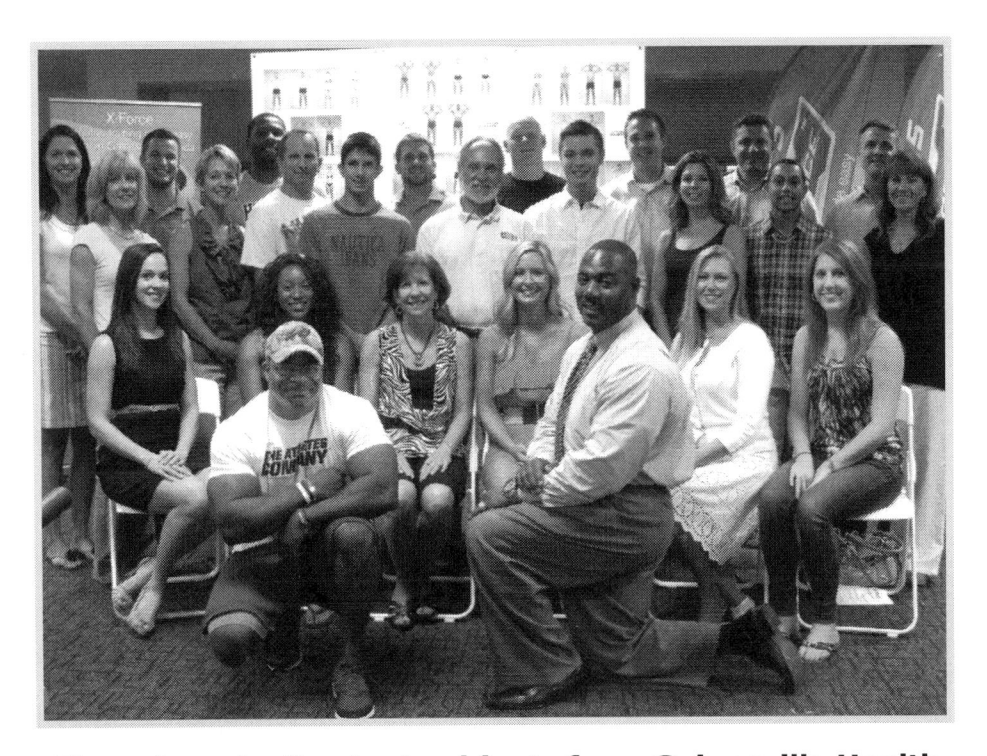

These twenty-five test subjects from Gainesville Health & Fitness Center have just finished one of my programs. The best before-and-after comparisons—some of which you will see in this book—are featured behind them.

Angel Rodriguez (see page 16): Of the 1,350 individuals I've trained at Gainesville Health & Fitness, eleven weighed more than 300 pounds when they started. But none of the 300-pounders ever reduced more than Angel Rodriguez. From a starting body weight of 281.5 pounds, Angel lost 121 pounds of fat. Can you imagine dropping 20 inches off your waist? That's exactly what Angel did. His workouts were amazing, as he is extremely strong and it shows throughout his physique. He also built 20.5 pounds of muscle.

Dana Crase (see page 17): A real-estate broker in central Florida, Dana is married with a couple of active grandkids. She lost almost 30 pounds of fat. Dana says, "My high-strung grandkids have their grandmother back in action. I can now run and tumble with them."

Both Dana and Angel challenge you to *Still Living Longer Stronger*.

Angel Rodriguez

Age 48, Height 5' 8"

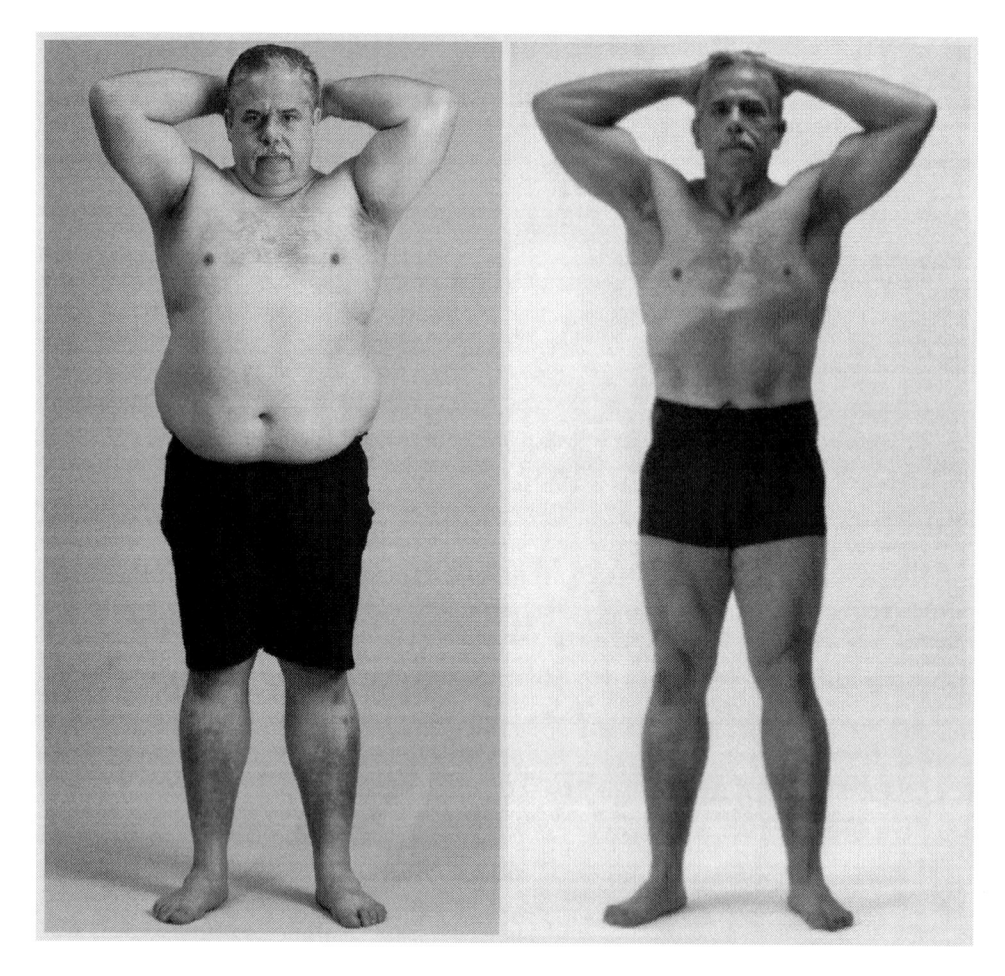

281.5 pounds   **181** pounds

After 30 weeks
121 pounds of fat loss, **20.125** inches off waist
20.5 pounds of muscle gain

"I drove to Miami and surprised my mother, who had not seen me in 7 months. She did *not* recognize me and started to call the cops. I had to assure her in Spanish that it was me, Angel, her transformed son."

Dana Crase

Age 63, Height 5' 1"

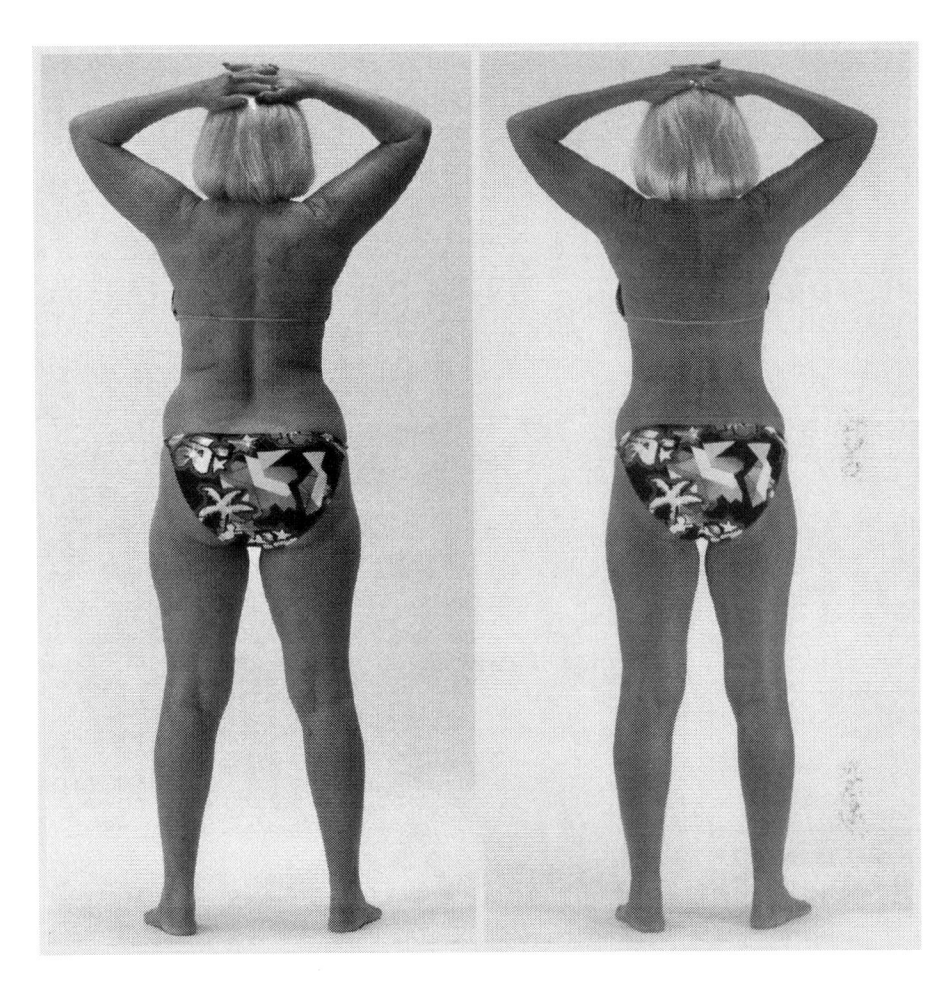

143 pounds   **122** pounds

After 18 weeks
28.7 pounds of fat loss, **6.5** inches off waist
7.7 pounds of muscle gain

"My husband saw me getting out of the pool from the backside in my new bikini and said he thought I was one of the college girls from the nearby apartments. As I faced him, we both smiled invitingly."

Fat: The Pluses

Fat is hated, yes. But you'd never want to eliminate it entirely from your body. Even the leanest people in the world have 5 percent of their body weight in fat. In fact, fat is a critical organ that has more influence on your body than you might think. For example:

- Fat cells pack together so efficiently that 20,000 calories weigh only 5 pounds.

- Fat cells produce warmth, insulate our organs, and serve as messengers for our immune system.

- Brain cells depend on fat. Parts of them are sheathed in a substance called myelin, which is made of fat.

- Fat cells make a hormone, leptin, that allows the brain to regulate appetite.

- Fat, through leptin, enhances the size and function of the brain.

- Fat influences sexual maturation, menstruation, and pregnancy. A certain amount of fat is needed to reproduce.

- Fat and bone influence each other reciprocally with hormones. Fat increases bone, and bone increases fat.

- Fat helps us sustain body functions during sickness and recovery.

Fat: The Minuses

You need a small amount of fat on your body. Too much, however, can cause problems.

- Fat cells have the unique ability to store fat, lots of it. Fat cells can expand their volume more than 1,000 times normal size by pushing other cell contents off to the side.

- When our fat cells are crowded, they no longer respond well to insulin, the hormone from the pancreas. The sugars and fats circulating in our bloodstreams start piling up in places they don't belong: the arteries, liver, and intestines.

- Abdominal fat is the most dangerous kind, and high levels of it correlate directly to diabetes, heart disease, and high cholesterol.

- As you reach your forties, the percentage of fat in your body increases and becomes more troublesome. Fat begins to accumulate on the belly and lower back of men and on the buttocks, thighs, and breasts of women.

- During your fifties and sixties, you are typically at your heaviest and have the most difficult time keeping fat in check.

- On all continents of the world, and in every race and culture, women store more fat than do men. The reasons: biology and hormones. Women are 80 percent of the fat-reduction market in the USA.

- Fat begets fat. Studies show that fat can grow right back after liposuction, and not necessarily in the same place it came from.

Still Living Longer 3 Stronger

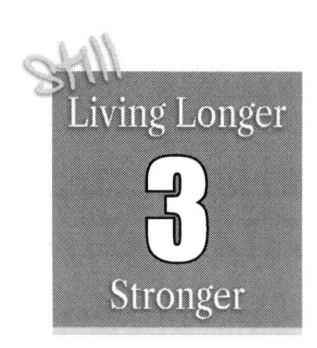

Biomarkers and Muscle

In March of 2023, I listened to an episode of a podcast called *Longevity by Design* in which Dr. William J. Evans was interviewed. Dr. Evans is an adjunct professor of medicine in the geriatrics program at Duke University and co-author of a best-selling book, *Biomarkers: 10 Determinants of Aging You Can Control.*

Up front, Dr. Evans pointed out that strength training is by far the most important thing we can do to delay aging. Stimulating muscle growth, he said, provides an answer to the age-old problems of fragility and infirmity.

"Over the last twenty-five years," Dr. Evans noted, "building muscle has become our number one priority in our nursing home studies. After only three months, we've seen a 100 to 200 percent increase in strength of men and women in their 90s. The before-and-after differences in posture, confidence, and performance are amazing."

I've been saying the same things as Dr. Evans for even longer than he has.

Dr. Peter Attia, in his 2023 book *Outlive: The Science and Art of Longevity*, discusses something many of us have witnessed: the slow death of someone we loved. Often our elders linger for years, alive but withered by illness in body, mind, or both.

A better idea, he writes, is to be active and progress to our deathbeds having lived fully to the end. Keeping your muscle mass sizable, hydrated, and strong is a big part of Dr. Attia's framework.

My friend Bill Kribs experienced such a life.

Bill Kribs: A Well-Armed Example

William R. Kribs, a real-estate developer in Orlando, Florida, lived down the street from my family and me. Beginning in 2014, I put him through fifty strength-training sessions spread over six months. During that time, Bill built 8.27 pounds of muscle. That's an average gain of 0.32 pounds of muscle per week for 26 consecutive weeks.

Several years later, to a group of older men who were cooling off after a Saturday workout in my home gym, Bill asserted the following: "To say that Ell's program has made a difference in my life is a huge understatement. In 2016, my daughter made an appointment for me to have a complete physical and mental evaluation by Orlando Health's Center for Aging. After several days of very thorough testing, they concluded I was perfectly healthy for a 70-year-old man. 'That's great,' I said, 'but you know what? I just celebrated my birthday: number 96.'"

Bill was born near St. Louis and was interested in music. At age 17, he played the saxophone and clarinet with great skill. Soon he was touring the country with some of the leading big bands of that era, such as Tommy Dorsey, Les and Larry Elkhart, and Sonny Durham. That continued for almost two decades.

I used to marvel as Bill told me stories of meeting and socializing with Frank Sinatra, Bing Crosby, Artie Shaw, Buddy Rich, Jo Stafford, Doris Day, and Peggy Lee.

Bill was married and fathered five children. He was an avid downhill skier as well as a sailboat racer. He owned and operated a small airplane and logged 4,000 flight hours. Bill had a Ford dealership in Orlando, but his real passion was real-estate development.

Bill never missed his Saturday workout session with his training buddies, and by the time he reached 100 years of age, he had recorded 300 workouts with me. Bill kept us all inspired with his strength, endurance, and independence.

Bill Kribs was a big believer in the idea that it's never too late to start strength training. Remember, he did not begin seriously building his muscles until he was 94, and it empowered his life.

Then suddenly, in August of 2021, Bill started losing his teeth and had difficulty eating. His body weight dropped by twenty pounds, most of which was muscle. He became dehydrated. He had trouble walking. He died quickly in December of 2021. He had lived a full, complete life. Bill was 101.

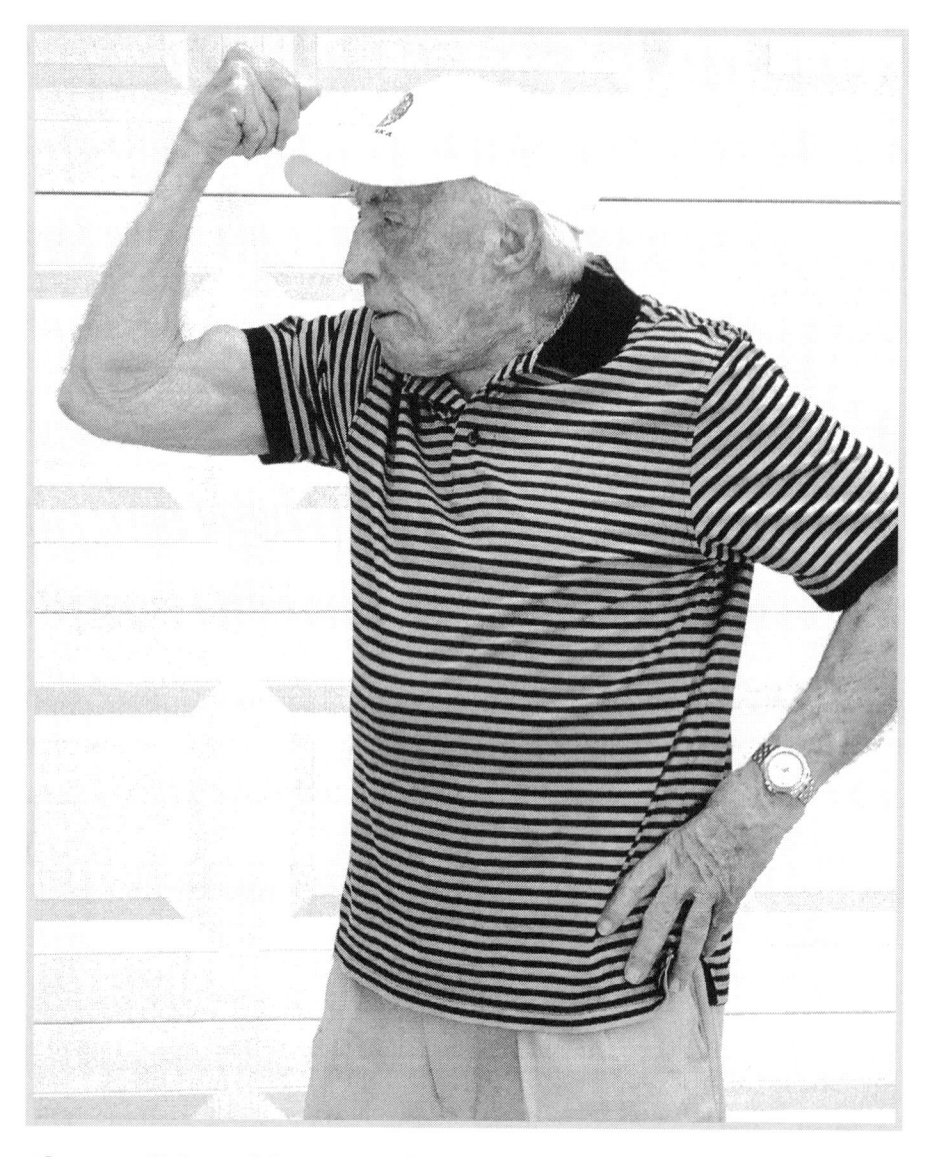

Starting well into his 90s, Bill Kribs built 11.35 pounds of solid muscle, which put his body weight at 158 pounds. He stood 5' 9" tall and had 14.5 percent body fat. Bill was a soft-spoken, gracious man—but he enjoyed impressing his close friends and selected visitors by contracting his biceps.

Your Destiny, Your Choice

Aging is too commonly associated with weakness, wrinkles, gray hair, retirement, forgetfulness, nursing homes, and death. Our concepts about age result from a complex mixture of prejudices, expectations, customs, and even legislation.

To better understand these concepts, scientists have targeted the aging process for detailed study. Although much research is yet to be done, there are still exciting findings to share.

Erosion of the human body is not inevitable, many scientists have concluded. Only death is unavoidable. Barring disease, many body functions decline very slowly with the proper exercise, nutrition, stimulation, and support.

This book will show you how to rebuild strength, health, and self-sufficiency and maintain them for the longest possible time. You can control your own destiny.

The Power of Strength Training

In the previously mentioned book *Biomarkers: 10 Determinants of Aging You Can Control*, Dr. Evans and Dr. Irwin Rosenberg report the findings of studies done at the USDA Human Nutrition Research Center on Aging at Tufts University. Their ten biomarkers, or physiological factors, associated with aging are as follows:

1. Muscle mass
2. Strength
3. Basal metabolic rate
4. Body fat percentage
5. Aerobic capacity
6. Blood-sugar tolerance
7. Cholesterol/HDL ratio
8. Blood pressure
9. Bone density
10. Internal temperature regulation

Not surprising to me is that each of these biomarkers is improved through the type of exercise recommended in *Still Living Longer Stronger*. Seventy years ago, this type of exercise was called weight-lifting. Later it was called weight training, strength training, and progressive-resistance exercise. Then, with the media's help, came the phrase "pumping iron." Although all these concepts apply, in my books and writings I've always been partial to the term *strength training*.

Strength training is also one of the keys to successful muscle building.

The Still Living Longer Stronger version of strength training is different from what you may have done in the past. It involves the lifting and lowering of weights (barbells, dumbbells, and machines), but each exercise requires slow, smooth movement—especially on the lowering. Slow and smooth movement, which eliminates excessive momentum, is much more effective than fast, jerky motion at stimulating your muscles to grow larger and stronger. You'll learn more about this in later chapters.

Here's how proper strength training affects each of the biomarkers listed above.

(1) **Muscle mass** and (2) **strength** go together. As your body adapts and lifts heavier and heavier weights, your muscles get stronger and larger. An average man, through proper strength training, can expect to increase his overall strength by 5 percent per week. Consequently, this 5 percent strength increase will add approximately one-half pound of muscle to his body.

Additional muscle elevates your (3) **basal metabolic rate**. Assuming your dietary calories per day remain unchanged, you'll notice a slight reduction in your (4) **body fat percentage**.

Proper strength training can boost your (5) **aerobic capacity** by improving your heart's ability to pump oxygen-rich blood to the working muscles.

Your (6) **blood-sugar tolerance**, or your body's ability to control the level of sugar in the blood, is enhanced by strength training. Generally, as people get older, they gradually lose muscle and gain fat. As a result, they needs more insulin—the hormone that removes sugar from the blood and transfers it to the body's tissues for fuel. Added muscle decreases the need for insulin and helps prevent adult-onset diabetes.

You've probably heard about the two kinds of cholesterol in our blood: HDL (high-density lipoprotein), which is protective, and LDL (low-density lipoprotein), which is problematic and often needs lowering. Several studies show that strength training and lowering body fat can raise blood levels of HDL as well as lowering total cholesterol. The (7) **cholesterol/HDL ratio** often significantly improves—which is an important factor in preventing heart attacks.

Along with controlling blood cholesterol, the exercise programs recommended in this book can help regulate (8) **blood pressure**. Learning to lift and lower heavy weights in the correct manner, however, is instrumental in avoiding problems and getting the best possible results. You'll get the most up-to-date instructions on how to do this in chapters 9 and 10.

Any time you build a muscle larger and stronger, you correspondingly increase your (9) **bone density**. Bone thinning, or osteoporosis, can be warded off with proper strength exercise.

Finally, strength training improves (10) **the body's ability to regulate its internal temperature**. Your body's built-in thermostat needs plenty of water to function correctly. Since your muscles are mostly composed of water, the six-week plan described in Part IV (chapter 15) of this book promotes superhydration each day. Plus, having more muscle in your body means you'll have a higher total water content, which helps regulate your internal temperature as well.

Say Yes to the *Still Living Longer Stronger* Plan

Can people in their 60s, 70s, or 80s who haven't been physically active for years really forge into this program and expect to hold back or even reverse the declines in their biomarkers? Yes! And will doing so reverse the effects of aging? Yes, again!

Throughout this book I'll present plenty of evidence to back up what I'm saying.

Still Living Longer 4 Stronger

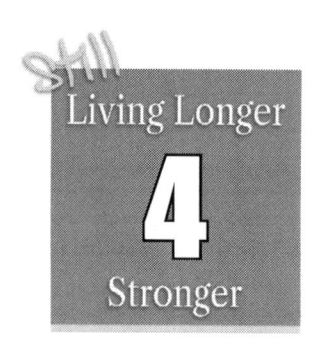

Disuse Atrophy and Creeping Obesity

Use it or lose it. That's the popular concept related to muscle that is taught in most physical education courses in the United States. The concept certainly applies to strength training. If you work harder this week than last week, your muscles grow slightly stronger. If you don't work as hard this week as you did the previous week, then a small amount of atrophy, or shrinkage, occurs.

Disuse Atrophy

A lot of the basic research on muscle atrophy was done by Dr. Gilbert Forbes of the Rochester School of Medicine. I first met Dr. Forbes during a 1975 Nautilus/West Point study. He helped with the body fat calculations of the cadets. At the time, Dr. Forbes was in the process of analyzing several decades' worth of data about how body composition changes as we age.

Dr. Forbes' full report was published in *Human Biology* in 1976. Basically, what he discovered was that between the ages of 20 and 50, average people who do not strength-train lose half a pound of muscle per year. This decline is called "disuse atrophy." Much of Dr. Forbes' original research has since been validated with the latest body-composition technology by Dr. William Evans and scientists at the Nutrition, Exercise Physiology, and Sarcopenia Laboratory at Tufts University in Boston.

Half a pound of muscle per year translates into slightly more than 22/100ths of an ounce per day, which seems insignificant. And it probably would be if not for the cumulative effect. Bit by bit, little by little, ounce by ounce, things add up. After a decade, it's 5 pounds. After thirty years, it's 15 pounds.

A loss of 15 pounds of muscle is nothing to laugh about. The next time you're at the supermarket, spend some time in the meat department. Pick up a 5-pound roast. Imagine holding three 5-pounders. That's approximately the space in your body that 15 pounds of your muscle occupies.

Of course, atrophy is not selective; it happens throughout your body, from all of your muscle areas. Perhaps two of the pounds shrink from each thigh, another pound from each buttock, a couple of pounds from your back, chest, and shoulders, a half-pound from each arm and each calf, and the remaining several pounds from around your lower back, midsection, and neck.

If that scenario is not enough to make you want to go and work out, then the next facts will for sure.

Creeping Obesity

Dr. Forbes also found that while average men and women are losing muscle ounce by ounce, they are also gaining fat—at triple the rate. That fat gain amounts to 1½ pounds each year, or 15 pounds per decade. That's a 45-pound fat gain over thirty years.

The losing and gaining process is so slow that it takes a decade or more to notice that something major is happening to your body—hence the term "creeping obesity."

Fat tissue is approximately 20 percent less dense than muscle, so it takes up 20 percent more space.

Next time you're at the supermarket, look at a 40-pound sack of dog food. That's how much space 45 pounds of fat takes up on your body. Get the picture?

The Effect on Metabolism

Your resting metabolism is the number of calories your body requires to operate in a relaxed state. Your brain and internal organs—especially your heart, lungs, liver, and kidneys—demand a lot of energy. But it's the skeletal muscles, which are 35 to 50 percent of your body weight, that have the most energy potential.

David Domash

Age 52, Height 5' 8"

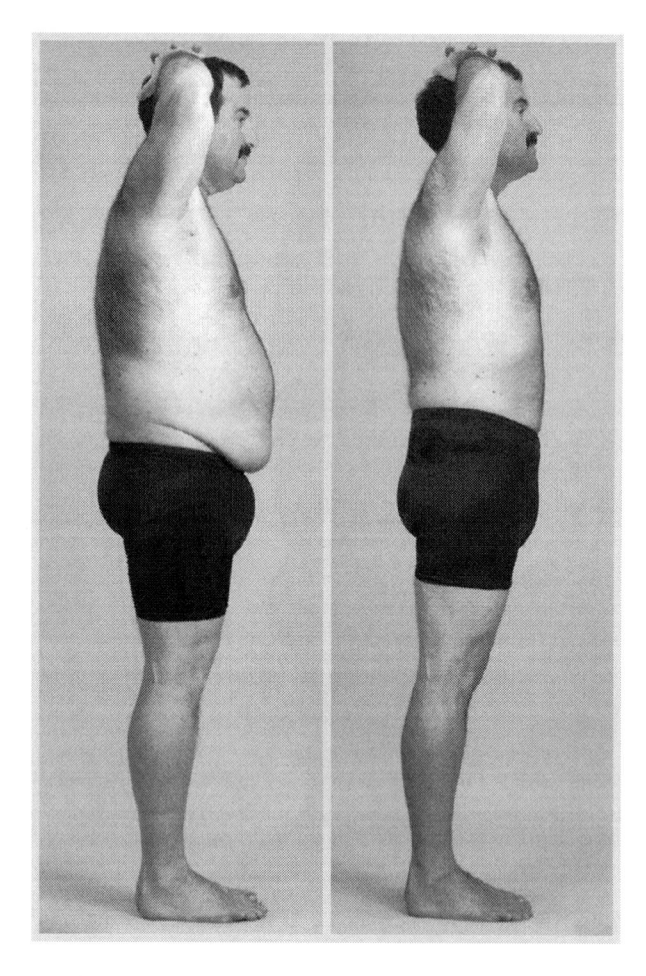

281.5 pounds   **174** pounds

After 12 weeks
41.4 pounds of fat loss, **9.75** inches off waist
7.4 pounds of muscle gain

"My energy is back to what it was in my 20s."

Lose a pound of muscle through atrophy, and your resting metabolic rate goes down approximately 37.5 calories per day. Add a pound through strength training, and your rate goes up by the same number.

A pound of fat tissue inside the human body also has a metabolic rate: 2 calories per day. Muscle is thus 18.75 times as metabolically active as the same amount of fat.

You've probably noticed that it is more difficult to shed excess fat than it used to be. Long-term metabolism studies reveal that an average person experiences a 0.5 percent reduction in resting metabolic rate each year between 20 and 50 years of age. The gradual loss of muscle mass each year is primarily responsible for this metabolic slowdown.

Insulin Sensitivity and Metabolic Health

Larger muscles also improve metabolic health. The reason: Muscles process glucose, and larger muscles increase insulin receptiveness.

Glucose, your body's primary energy source, comes from the foods you eat. When your blood glucose goes up, it signals your pancreas to release a hormone called insulin. Insulin regulates the amount of glucose in the blood.

When you build muscle mass, the muscle cells use more glucose with less need for insulin. Less insulin is positive. Too much can cause insulin resistance, which is when cells aren't as responsive to insulin and blood glucose rises to dangerous levels.

The other side of insulin resistance is insulin sensitivity. When you are more insulin-sensitive, your body processes glucose more efficiently, with less insulin. Research shows that strength training and muscle building improve insulin sensitivity and metabolic health.

Muscle Your Fat Away

Certainly, controlling dietary calories is an important aspect of combating creeping obesity. But equally important is the building, or rebuilding, of muscle mass.

Don't let your fat cells grow while your muscles wither. It's time to muscle your fat away. My 10-10-10 method of strength training will put you in the driver's seat.

Still Living Longer 5 Stronger

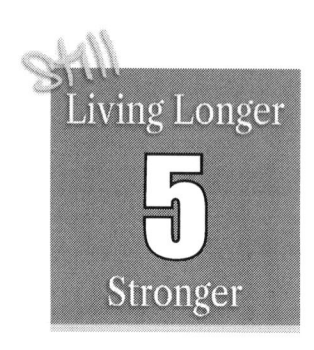

Building Muscle and Losing Fat
. . . Simultaneously

The first half of this chapter is for women. The second half deals with men.

Components of Body Weight

Stepping on the bathroom scale is a daily ritual for many women. There is a prevalent belief that appearance and well-being depend on body weight.

Your body weight is simply an estimate of the shape, condition, and appearance of your figure. To be more meaningful, your body weight must be separated into four components.

The four major components of your body weight are as follows:

- Bone
- Organs
- Muscle
- Fat

Your bones make up from 12 to 14 percent of your body weight, and your organs (including skin) occupy from 25 to 30 percent of it. Those items don't change significantly as you age, but the remaining two—muscle and fat—do. Your percentages of muscle and fat are critical to this discussion because they are the components you can change through diet and exercise.

Much of the Still Living Longer Stronger challenge centers around an understanding of muscle and fat . . . or more specifically, optimizing your muscle/fat ratio.

The Average Woman

Over the past forty years, I've done body composition measurements on more than a thousand women. In addition, I've talked with and observed the figure problems of thousands more. The following chart is representative of the average woman that I've worked with. Let me describe and illustrate her body composition from age 14 to 50.

Muscle/Fat Ratio Changes
Average Woman As She Ages

Age	14	20	30	40	50
Body weight (lbs)	130	136	146	156	166
Muscle (lbs)	51	48	43	38	33
Fat (lbs)	24	33	48	63	78
Percent body fat	18.5	24.3	32.9	40.4	47

From ages 14 to 50, women see their muscle mass decline and their fat increase.

Between the ages of 14 and 50, the average woman who does not do strength-training exercise loses 0.5 pounds of muscle per year and gains 1.5 pounds of fat per year.

My measurements and observations show that the average female is generally at her peak muscularly at age 14. At a height of 5 feet 5 inches and a body weight of 130 pounds, her muscle weighs 51 pounds and her fat weighs 24 pounds. Her muscle/fat ratio is 51/24, or 2.13/1. In other words, she has 2.13 pounds of muscle for each pound of fat. Because of this high ratio of muscle to fat, her body is firm, hard, and well defined.

With each passing year, however, she loses 0.5 pounds of muscle and gains 1.5 pounds of fat. The specifics are listed in the chart.

The Average Woman, Age 50

At age 50, after having and raising an average of 2.2 children, she weighs 166 pounds, which is a gain of 36 pounds of body weight since age 14. More specifically, her muscle has decreased by 18 pounds while her fat has increased by 54 pounds. Furthermore, her percentage of body fat has gone from 18.5 to 47—a 154 percent increase.

What causes this influx of fat and gradual loss of muscle? The primary reasons are too many dietary calories, faulty eating habits, lack of proper exercise, pregnancy and childbirth, and the natural aging process.

Melissa Norman

Age 48, Height 5' 2"

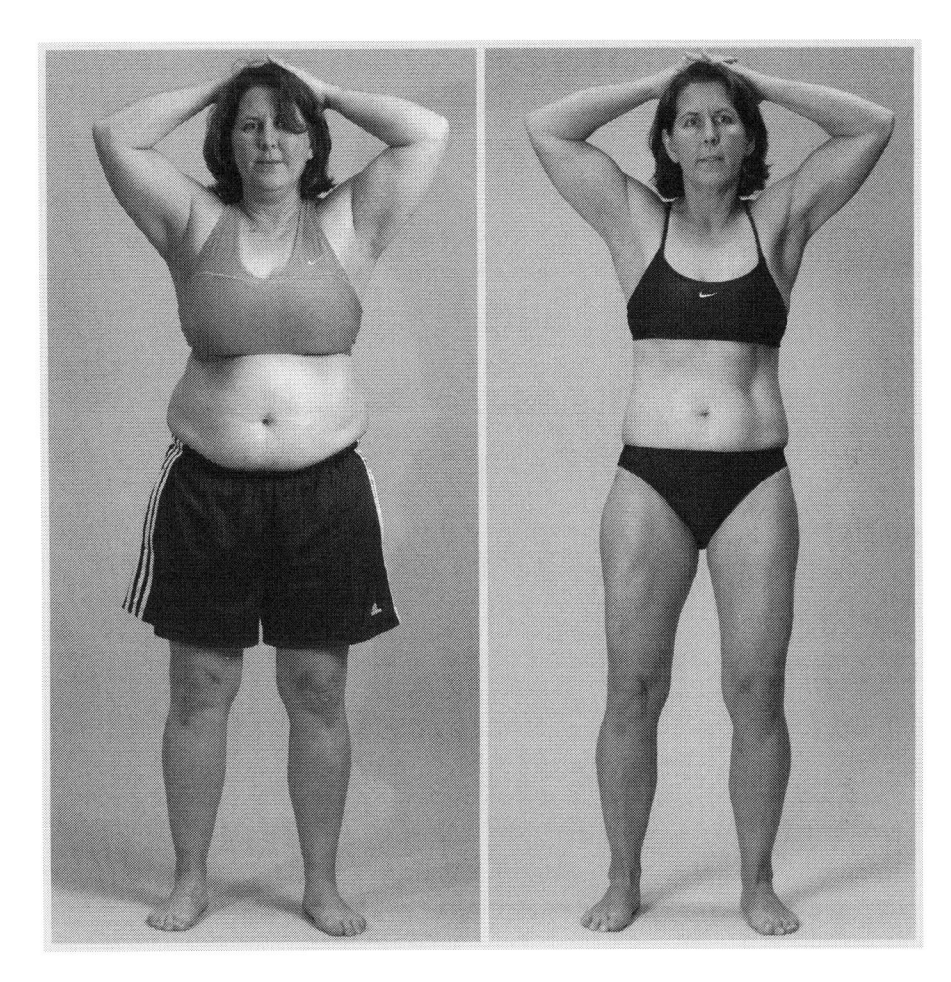

173 pounds   **129.4** pounds

After 18 weeks
52.2 pounds of fat loss, **12.625** inches off waist, **6** inches off hips
8.6 pounds of muscle gain

"My overall results were in reverse to Dr. Darden's Average Woman as She Ages chart. My fat went down and my muscle went up— both significantly. My 130-pound body weight today is what I weighed in high school. I almost feel like a teenager again."

More Muscle, Less Fat

The average woman in her 30s, 40s, or 50s needs significantly less fat and more muscle. The average woman needs what *Still Living Longer Stronger* has to offer.

All the causative factors listed in the last section, except for the aging process, are subject to your control. With discipline, patience, and the guidelines presented in this book, you can successfully lose fat and build muscle at the same time. Doing so will have a significant effect on your muscle/fat ratio and an enormous effect on the appearance of your midsection, hips, thighs, and upper body.

The Average Man Needs the Living Longer Stronger Program

The average man I've trained over the years is 6 feet tall and weighs 175 pounds at age 20. His body weight is composed of 12 percent bone, 15 percent fat, 47 percent muscle, and 26 percent organs, skin, and other.

Using the statistics from the last chapter, let's fast-forward twenty years.

At age 40, our average man has lost 10 pounds of muscle and gained 30 pounds of fat. His percentage of body fat has gone from 15 to 28.85, and his muscle has decreased from 47 to 37.05 percent. As a result, his body weight has risen from 175 to 195.

In twenty years, our average man has gone from a decent physical condition to being overfat, under-muscled, and out of shape. Furthermore, he is now at higher risk for specific medical conditions, such as high blood pressure, kidney disease, diabetes mellitus, stroke, and impairment of heart function.

In Six Weeks or Longer

What our average man needs is the Still Living Longer Stronger plan that is described in Part IV. In only six weeks, he can lose 21 pounds of fat while simultaneously building 4 pounds of muscle. As a result, his body fat percentage will decrease from 28.85 to 19.80, and his muscle will increase from 37.05 to 42.84 percent.

Although he has not quite recaptured his 20-year-old body, he is close. If he continues the program for another six weeks, his 40-something physique will be in better shape than it was twenty years earlier. And his risks for the listed medical conditions will be significantly reduced. In my programs over the last few years, I've seen some amazing results occur.

Some men may require only six weeks. Others may need 12 or even 18 weeks.

A Few Examples

In my programs, I've seen some amazing results. As examples, I'm listing five women and five men:

- Phyllis Hildebrand, a 54-year-old accountant, lost 27¾ pounds of fat and built 4¼ pounds of muscle in 10 weeks.
- Carolyn Cannon, a 64-year-old schoolteacher, lost 47 pounds of fat and built 5 pounds of muscle in 20 weeks.
- Barrie Gaffney, a 41-year-old mother of three, lost 22½ pounds of fat and built 4 pounds of muscle in 6 weeks.
- Claude Howell, a 53-year-old secretary, lost 21½ pounds of fat and built 5½ pounds of muscle in 12 weeks.
- Dr. Paula Golombek, a 51-year-old university professor, lost 32 pounds of fat and built 7¾ pounds of muscle in 18 weeks.
- Richard Ives, a 47-year-old businessman, lost 24¾ pounds of fat and built 4 pounds of muscle in 32 days.
- Ron Travis, a 46-year-old businessman, lost 21¾ pounds of fat and built 5 pounds of muscle in 32 days.
- Ted Blake, a 41-year-old plumber, lost 42½ pounds of fat and built 3½ pounds of muscle in 70 days.
- Bob Smith, a 51-year-old schoolteacher, lost 80 pounds of fat and built 19 pounds of muscle in 80 days.
- Storm Roberts, a 61-year-old radio host, lost 65½ pounds of fat and built 10¾ pounds of muscle in 105 days.

Building from Fat

How does your body build muscle on a lower-calorie diet? It draws most of the chemicals necessary for growth from your fat cells. Since a pound of fat supplies 3,500 calories and a pound of muscle contains only 600 calories, it's possible to build 5 pounds of muscle from 1 pound of fat. Over 70 percent of muscle is water, and water is void of calories. Fat, on the other hand, is mostly fat—which is composed of greasy, waxy lipid material.

One more fact about fat and muscle will be of interest to you.

Scientists have taken samples of fat and muscle from throughout the human body and counted the number of cells. Although this research is still in its infancy and depends on extrapolation, the average man appears to have approximately 25 billion fat cells and 10 billion muscle cells. Women have more fat cells and less muscle cells than do men.

Each of these microscopically small cells has the capacity to inflate or deflate. Obviously, it is to your advantage to inflate your muscle cells and deflate your fat cells.

Women and Men: What to Expect

On average, what can a woman and a man in their second middle age—between 45 and 70—expect from the Still Living Longer Stronger (SLLS) strength training program? They can anticipate the following:

- A 5 percent increase in strength per week, or at least per two weeks, in all the basic exercises. For example, if you can perform the standing biceps curl with a 30-pound barbell for 10 repetitions during week one, then during week two, you should be able to do the same number of repetitions with 32½ pounds. At the end of six weeks, you should be able to curl 40 pounds for 10 repetitions, which translates to an approximate 30-percent improvement in your biceps' strength.

- A ½-pound overall gain of muscle mass per week. My testing and experience over the years have shown that the average 45- to 70-year-old person can build 3 to 4 pounds of muscle during the initial six-week strength training program.

The typical 45- to 70-year-old individual can continue strength and muscle mass increases for another six to twelve weeks. Naturally, the rate of gain decreases with progress. But the man who is consistent with the discipline can expect to double his muscular strength and add 10 to 12 pounds of muscle to his body during the first nine to twelve months. The average woman can expect about 25 percent less muscle gain.

Combine this predicted muscle gain with a 20- to 40-pound loss of fat, and your own mother may not recognize you at first glance.

Yes, you can build muscle and lose fat—and you can do both together.

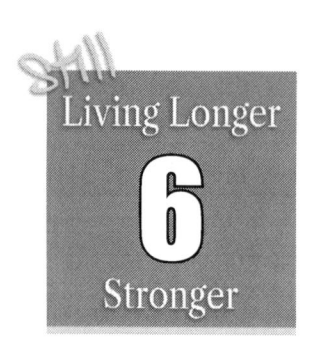

Not Just Stronger, But Enduring and Flexible

The three elements of well-rounded fitness are muscular strength, cardiovascular endurance, and joint flexibility. The Still Living Longer Stronger program incorporates all three into one potent package.

There is no need for multiple programs. In the past, books started out as handwritten manuscripts, which were then passed to a typist, followed by typesetter, and then a technician who made plates for a printing press. Now, virtually all those steps can be performed on a single computer. Our exercise technology has likewise advanced to the point of time-saving efficiency.

Examine these fringe benefits of the strength-building strategy of the SLLS program.

Cardiovascular Endurance

Your cardiovascular system is comprised of the heart, arteries, capillaries, and veins. Your heart is a special four-chambered muscle that serves as a storage tank and a pump for moving blood through your body. Arteries are the tubular vessels that carry blood away from your heart. Capillaries are tiny single-layer vessels in the tissues themselves where the actual exchange of oxygen, nutrients, and waste materials takes place. Your capillaries then connect with a system of small veins, which gradually become larger as they return blood to your lungs for re-oxygenation and then back to the heart for recirculation.

Improving cardiovascular endurance requires exercise, but not just any exercise. Specifically:

- The exercise must be hard enough to elevate your heart rate (measured in beats per minute) to 60 to 85 percent of your body's maximum capacity.
- That elevated heart rate must be sustained for a minimum of 10 minutes.
- Such exercise should be repeated at least three times a week.

First, estimate your maximum heart rate by subtracting your age from 220.

$$220 - \underbrace{}_{\text{your age}} = \underbrace{}_{\substack{\text{your maximum} \\ \text{heart rate}}} \text{bpm}$$

Then calculate the range for your target heart rate by multiplying as follows:

$$\underbrace{}_{\substack{\text{your maximum} \\ \text{heart rate}}} \times\ 0.6 = \underbrace{}_{\substack{\text{your } \textit{minimum} \\ \text{target heart rate}}} \text{bpm}$$

$$\underbrace{}_{\substack{\text{your maximum} \\ \text{heart rate}}} \times\ 0.85 = \underbrace{}_{\substack{\text{your } \textit{maximum} \\ \text{target heart rate}}} \text{bpm}$$

For example, if you are 60, your estimated maximum heart rate is 220 minus 60, or 160 beats per minute. To improve cardiovascular endurance, your workout should enable you to maintain a heart rate of 60 to 85 percent of that number, or 96 to 136 beats per minute.

Strength and Cardiovascular Endurance

Next, let's address that second requirement for improving cardiovascular endurance: maintaining your target heart rate for at least

10 minutes. Typically, we think of jogging, swimming, stair-climbing, and cycling as activities for improving cardiovascular endurance. And they can—but so can a well-devised strength training workout.

It doesn't matter to your heart which muscles are being exercised to elevate your heart rate to the desired level. Working your arms has the same effect on your heart as working your legs, provided the total amount of work and the pace are the same.

The key to maintaining that target heart rate during strength training is not to rest too long between exercises: usually no more than 15 to 30 seconds. Your workout should be organized into a sequence of exercises that you initiate one right after another. This style of training is like the no-huddle offense you now see in college and professional football. In other words, after each exercise, get to the next one as if time were running out.

By maintaining an elevated heart rate, a no-huddle circuit of strength training increases not just strength but also cardiovascular endurance.

Not Just Stronger, But Enduring and Flexible | 41

Dr. Boyd Welsch

Age 68, Height 6' 1"

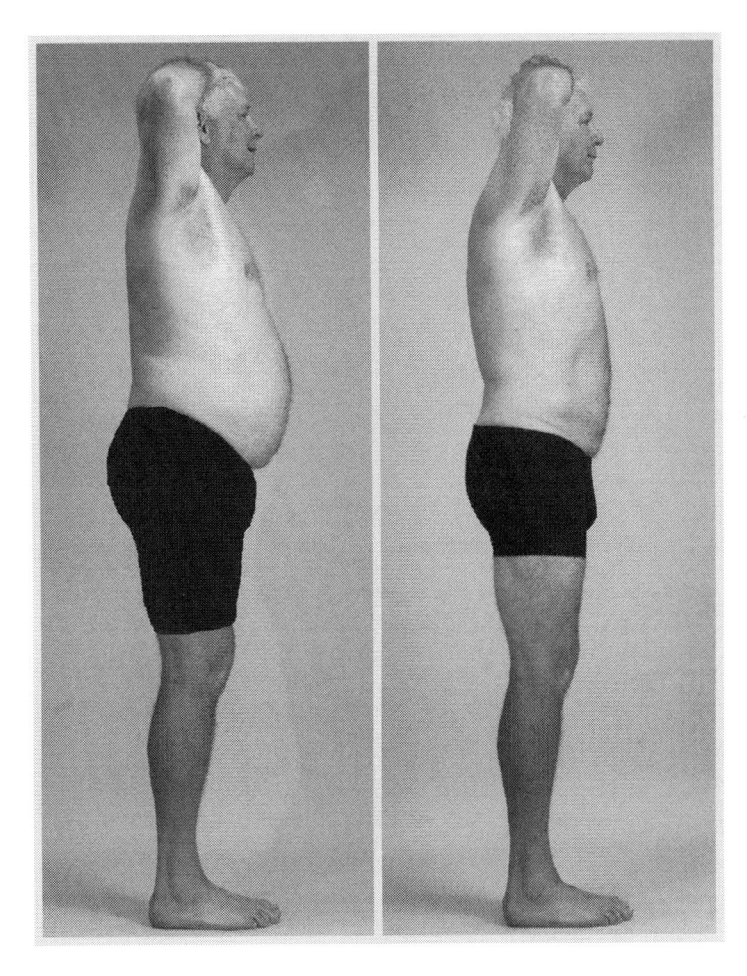

262 pounds   **223.5** pounds

After 12 Weeks
49.27 pounds of fat loss, **11.25** inches off waist
10.77 pounds of muscle gain

"This has truly been a life-altering experience for me."

Joint Flexibility

Flexibility is the range and ease of movement of a body part around a joint.

When your joints are flexible, you can bend forward and touch your toes while keeping your legs stiff, and you can reach behind your back, turn your head, and stretch comfortably into an assortment of positions. Most of second-middle-agers remember playing a game called Twister. They probably also shimmied under a bamboo pole in a dance called the Limbo.

Flexibility is essential to the maintenance and safekeeping of joints, muscles, and connective tissues. Anatomically, the limiting factors in flexibility are tendons, ligaments, muscle fibers, and muscle fascia or sheath. Tendons are not meant to be stretched. Ligaments adapt to slight stretching, but once stretched, they will not return to normal length. Muscle fibers, on the other hand, have great capacity for stretching. The muscle fascia—the connective tissue sheath that encloses groups of muscle fibers—is stretchable also.

With proper exercise, your muscles and muscle fascia will adapt by stretching and becoming more flexible.

Full-Range Strength and Flexibility

The stretching exercises in this book are designed to increase your flexibility. In order to trigger the adaptation process that produces enhanced flexibility, a stretching exercise has to meet certain requirements:

- The exercise needs to be done smoothly—never by a sudden force or a jerk.
- The exercise must cover the full range from maximum stretch to full-muscular contraction. (This is achieved progressively, not all at once.)
- The stretch needs to be done "under load." This means the targeted muscle must be not only stretched, but also challenged to lift a weight that is heavy for it.

The SLLS program will teach you to stretch your muscles smoothly, under load, progressing gradually to the full range of motion. The full-range element of it—moving from maximum stretch to full-muscular contraction–qualifies the endeavor to also be termed flexibility training.

A Potent Package

I used to not know better. I used to believe that it was necessary to have separate routines for muscular strength, cardiovascular endurance, and joint flexibility. I now know that having separate routines is wasteful and inefficient.

Still Living Longer Stronger acknowledges muscular strength as the central factor of fitness and promotes strength training as the best form of exercise. But it does this in a way that also builds cardiovascular endurance and enhances flexibility—leveraging new research to save you time and help you succeed faster than before.

Proper strength training is indeed a potent package.

Why Only One Set of a Few Exercises?

Back in my competitive bodybuilding days (primarily the 1960s), I used to do two to three sets of most exercises. I would spend at least an hour doing a workout, training five days a week. So, my multi-set workouts required at least five hours per week.

When I entered graduate school at Florida State University in 1968, I had to reduce my time doing strength training and bodybuilding workouts due to work and study commitments. I went from five days a week of training to four days and then three days per week. Instead of five hours per week, I was doing three hours per week.

Guess what? My overall results improved. From a 40 percent reduction in my exercise time per week, my results were better.

Then, I met Arthur Jones, the man who invented Nautilus exercise equipment, and he convinced me to train even less. Instead of one-hour workouts, I applied 30-minute ones. In other words, I cut my workout in half.

The key, according to Jones, was the intensity, focus, and form you put into each exercise—not the total amount of time. In fact, as you increase the intensity, focus, and form, you *must* resort to a shorter workout time.

In other words, *quality* is more important than *quantity*.

When I completed my graduate work at Florida State University in 1972, I immediately took a job as director of research for Arthur Jones's Nautilus Sports/Medical Industries. Not only was I interested in developing exercise machines and marketing them, but I wanted to determine the best ways to workout on the equipment.

In the bodybuilding community, guys want to train more, not less. Nautilus could have sold more machines by simply saying: "Unfortunately, the Nautilus machines require more sets per exercise and more time in the gym." That would have made better sense to most strength athletes. But instead, all the Nautilus research revealed just the opposite: *less exercise—but with greater attention given to intensity, focus, and form*—was better.

Throughout the 1970s and 1980s, we continued to research and push the results (see sidebar below). Nautilus Fitness Centers flourished, and a strength-training boom was occurring.

What we discovered at Nautilus Sports/Medical Industries was that a person's potential strength did not increase in proportion to his or her recovery ability. Most untrained people have the capacity to increase their strength by 300 percent. But their recovery ability amounts to an improvement of only 50 percent. Very simply, this means: *the stronger a person becomes, the less exercise he or she needs* to continue in a progressive manner.

In reality, however, most trainees do the opposite: the stronger they get, the more exercise they perform. Thus, they reach a certain level of strength, and even though they may stimulate their muscle to get stronger, they never *permit* this to happen. They seldom do less.

My 10-10-10 method helps you even more because it focuses on the lowering phase, the most productive part of each repetition. And it's much safer than traditional multiple-set ways of training.

After more than sixty years of personal experience in exercise and bodybuilding, plus the supervised training of thousands of test subjects and the publishing of more than fifty books, here's my bottom line:

One set of eight exercises, performed twice a week, is all you need for the best results.

Strength-Training Research

To explore the logical thinking plus the research behind the one-set guideline, see the following books and articles.

- *Nautilus Training Principles, Bulletin No. 1* (1970) by Arthur Jones.
- "Total Conditioning: The West Point Study" (1975) by James A. Peterson.
- *Strength-Training Principles* (1977) by Ellington Darden.
- *The Nautilus Bodybuilding Book* (1982) by Ellington Darden.
- "Alterations in Strength and Maximum Oxygen Uptake Consequent to Nautilus Circuit Weight Training" (1985) by Stephen Messier and Mary Dill.
- *Strength Fitness* (1995) by Wayne Westcott.
- *The New High Intensity Training* (2004) by Ellington Darden.

II

REEXAMINING STRENGTH TRAINING AND NUTRITION

Still Living Longer 7 Stronger

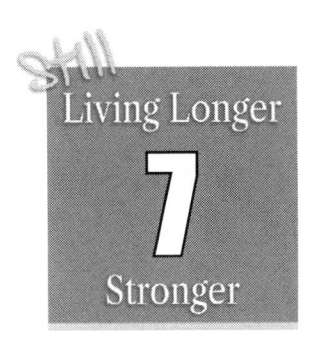

The Negative Awakening, 10-10-10, and Lift & Lower-Slower

From age 15 to 30, I was seriously interested in bodybuilding and weight training. I exercised to have a bigger, better-shaped, and stronger body. Furthermore, I competed successfully in more than fifty Amateur Athletic Union (AAU) bodybuilding contests.

During that time, from 1958 to 1973, I read a lot of what were called "muscle magazines." The publications that I so eagerly read, reread, and digested had titles such as *Strength & Health*, *Muscular Development*, *Mr. America*, and *Muscle Builder*. The most interesting magazine—when you could find it on the newsstand, which was not often—was called *IronMan*. Thus, I became an *IronMan* subscriber in 1968.

IronMan, 1972

One day, I picked up the latest issue of *IronMan* from the mailbox and thumbed through it quickly. *Hold it!*—something on pages 30 and 31 caught my eye . . . and it was the word *negative*. The article was "Accentuate the NEGATIVE." I had read other articles by the same writer, Arthur Jones, but this is the one I remember the best, even after more than fifty years.

Toward the end of the article, Jones challenged readers: "Start thinking in terms of NOT how much you can lift, but rather—how much you can lower." No lifter I knew of, nor read about, had ever talked about how much he could lower. It was always how much they could lift.

That single article greatly influenced me and thousands of other fitness-minded people.

From a scientific viewpoint, lifting a weight involves *concentric* muscle action, and lowering a weight requires *eccentric* muscle action. Jones thought those labels were confusing, so he used *positive* to mean concentric and *negative* to mean eccentric. As a result of Jones's writings, *positive* and *negative* are now a normal part of the bodybuilding and weight training lexicon.

I had met Jones two years earlier, in 1970, when he was in the process of starting Nautilus Sports/Medical Industries. Jones and Nautilus had begun manufacturing and marketing Nautilus strength-training machines, which were a radical departure from traditional barbells and dumbbells. At that time I was in Tallahassee, Florida, working on a PhD in exercise science at Florida State University. I visited Jones several times at his headquarters in Lake Helen, Florida, about 225 miles south of Tallahassee.

I got along well with Jones, which was something many people did not do, and I even told him I wanted to work for Nautilus when I finished my research at Florida State. Two more occurrences soon reinforced that conviction.

A Muddy Experience

During one of my visits with Arthur, I showed him an article I'd written about exercising in a mud pit in Waco, Texas. A man I met in Waco had dug a rectangular pit, lined it with concrete, and filled it with river-bottom clay from the nearby Brazos River. You stood in the clay, which was almost chin-deep, between a couple of tightly stretched horizontal ropes that held you in place. The clay provided resistance against various body movements. Imagine doing open-handed curls underwater; clay supplied a harder version of the same challenge. I had trained in the mud pit several times, and I showed Jones my article about what it was like.

Jones quickly analyzed the movements and pointed out something to me that I had not considered. "The problem with mud resistance," he noted, "is that it provides no negative work. And without negative work, an exercise is of limited value."

Instantly, I realized Jones was right. Imagine again the example of doing open-handed curls against the resistance of liquid clay. Once you contract your biceps and get to the top of the curl, there's little negative resistance on the lowering to challenge your triceps. If you really force yourself to extend your arm as fast as you can, you'll be working your triceps, but nothing says you *have* to do that. Mud (and water) exercise movements basically provide positive-only work.

Munich, 1972

A month after I read Arthur Jones's article "Accentuate the NEGATIVE," I was in Munich, Germany, attending the scientific congress that preceded the 1972 Olympic Games there. In one of the sessions, Finnish physiologist Dr. Paavo Komi described how he had trained a small group of Scandinavian weightlifters by having them lower—not lift—heavier-than-normal barbells from overhead to the floor. He was confident that his negative training would provide these weightlifters with an edge in their approaching Olympic competitions. Several days later, three of Dr. Komi's athletes won medals: two bronzes and one gold.

I told Dr. Komi I was interested in his ongoing research and wanted to talk with him more in the future. I also mentioned that I would soon be working with Arthur Jones of Nautilus Sports/Medical Industries. Dr. Komi shared with me he'd experimented with using various hydraulic machines to help with the lifting of extremely heavy barbells for his athletes, but the machines had been problematic to use.

From Prototype to Production

When I flew back to Florida from Germany, I phoned Jones and told him about Dr. Komi and his research with negative work.

"Bring those reports down to me," Jones replied.

I knew it would be a month before I could break away to visit Jones, so I mailed Komi's research study to him for his inspection.

When I finally got to Lake Helen, I was surprised to find that Jones and his prototyping team had built five functioning machines, which he called Omni. The Omni was a big, bulky contraption. It had a foot pedal that allowed the user to leg-press the loaded weight stack to the top position. Then you could grasp the movement arm with your hands and perform the negative portion of the specific exercise with your arms and involved upper-body muscles.

The advantage of the Omni was that it allowed you to work your upper-body muscles with negative movements using a much heavier weight than you could normally lift. Believe me, this negative training concept worked—well enough that Nautilus manufactured and sold hundreds of Omni machines for a growing market.

Jones always pushed the idea of performing each repetition in a smooth, slow manner, with no sudden movements. Performing negative exercise at a steady pace, he said, assured more complete exercise of the muscles because it provided more thorough stimulation of the muscle fibers. This was in contrast to our natural inclination to jerk the weight up and then drop it, the way a great deal of lifting was performed then and even now.

Negative Training Drawbacks

There are some problems inherent in negative training. First you can't work your legs in this manner—and trying to use your arms to assist your legs doesn't work well. What you can do is get a couple of strong training partners to help you do the lifting of the movement arm on the various leg exercises, such as the leg curl and the leg press, as you use a heavier-than-normal amount of resistance. Your spotters must be careful at the top to transfer the load smoothly to your legs. Such lifting soon becomes tedious for even the most motivated assistants.

Second is the problem of your own strength. You will become very strong, and quickly, from negative work. As a result, you may need another strong spotter to help you do the foot-pedal lifting. Again, that usually leads to an ongoing situation of trying to find a willing spotter.

Third is the problem of accurately judging the intensity of your negative repetitions. You can easily lapse into resting too long between repetitions.

A lag time of only three seconds allows your muscles a significant degree of recovery. Too much recovery means you are lowering the intensity, and you won't make gains in strength.

Fourth, resting too long between repetitions can actually be dangerous. A three-second, or longer, rest or lag time between repetitions means that you are performing a series of single-attempt efforts. Such lifting can lead to poor form and possibly injury.

The Machine Stalemate

As the years went by, Jones was in a quandary. He made many attempts to design machines with significantly more resistance on the negative stroke than on the positive stroke. First was the Omni machine, which supplied a foot pedal to lift a heavier-than-normal resistance with the legs so the user could then lower it with the arms. Eventually he designed electrically powered machines with servomotors that could be computer-programmed to supply more resistance on the negative. Jones's endeavors provided benefits, but the machines were cumbersome and complex.

Jones sold Nautilus in 1986, and he retired from his follow-up company, MedX, in 1996. He died in 2007 having never solved the problems of constructing a simple and reasonably affordable exercise machine that could provide more negative than positive resistance.

You had to really understand what you were doing with negative training for it to be beneficial for more than two months.

X-Force Emerges

In 2008, I got a phone call from a distributor of Nautilus equipment in Scandinavia. His name was Mats Thulin, and I remembered having met him in 1980 at a Nautilus seminar in Florida. Thulin invited me to travel to Stockholm, Sweden, and try his new machines, which he called X-Force. A month later, I was in Stockholm having an X-Force workout. I was more than impressed, as I could almost instantly feel the effect of negative training on my involved muscles.

The ingenuity of X-Force is a tilting weight stack that unloads the positive phase, then overloads the negative phase. In a series of fourteen strength training machines, X-Force supplies negative-accentuated exercise—40 percent more negative resistance than positive—with no need for assistants. Instead of searching for ways to add resistance to the negative, which was the strategy Jones and others had chosen, Thulin figured out a way to subtract weight from the positive. This was a brilliant step forward in the advancement of strength training machines.

But the machines were not without problems. For one thing, they were expensive: $12,000 for each one, meaning a complete line of the fourteen machines cost $168,000. Each contained a servomotor that required an electrical connection. Once in use, a machine needed maintenance, which could be time-consuming and required specific knowledge, creating even more expense.

Despite the problems, I had to get my hands on a set of X-Force equipment for my research. It took three years for me to work out a deal between Mats Thulin of X-Force and Joe Cirulli of Gainesville Health & Fitness. The X-Force equipment arrived in Gainesville, Florida, in January of 2012. By December, some ten months later, I had supervised the training of 145 people—and the results, both in fat loss and in muscle gain, were significantly better than any similar groups I had trained in my fifty years of doing research.

A Close Look at the Negative

Because of its cost, X-Force has not become a household name in the United States. X-Force is in only three American cities: Gainesville, Tampa, and Philadelphia. My challenge, since I had experienced and observed the muscle-building results, was to figure out how to adapt conventional strength training machines to simulate X-Force results. How could negative training be accomplished with traditional machines? Over the next year, through experimentation and testing, I came up with a technique that supplied 80 percent of the strength-building results of using an X-Force machine.

Initially, I tried a technique I called 30-30-30. It involved a slow 30-second negative, followed by a 30-second positive, then a final 30-second negative.

Next, I reduced the time for each phase to 15 seconds and called it 15-15-15, plus 8 to 12 normal reps at the end.

Then, I moved the normal reps to the middle of two 30-second negatives. That technique was called 30-10-30.

Finally, I shortened 30-10-30 to something that seemed ideal for older men and women. I called it 10-10-10.

The 10-10-10 Method

10-10-10 stands for a slow **10**-second negative (lowering) repetition, followed immediately by **10** faster positive/negative repetitions with controlled turnarounds (going from negative to positive or positive to negative), and finally another **10**-second negative repetition. The entire set takes approximately 50 seconds.

Here's an exercise, the biceps curl for your upper arms, that you can try with a couple of dumbbells to get acquainted with the 10-10-10 method. Use 10-pound dumbbells if you are a woman, 15-pound dumbbells if you are a man. You'll also need a clock with a second hand in plain sight nearby.

Grasp the dumbbells and stand with your arms hanging by your sides. Turn your hands so the dumbbells are longways and your thumbs are to the outside. With your elbows at your side, curl the weights to the top. Pause. You are now ready to begin 10-10-10. Look closely at the second hand on the clock, and begin lowering the dumbbells as the second hand crosses 12.

Progress smoothly at 2, 3, and 4 seconds. Try to be halfway down, where your forearms are parallel to the floor, at the 5-second mark. Breathe and continue to 8, 9, and 10 seconds.

At the bottom of the 10-second lowering, switch to doing 10 faster positive-negative repetitions. Take about 1 second on each positive and 2 seconds on each negative movement.

After your last positive repetition, do a finishing 10-second negative, with the same second-by-second guides. You should be able to feel the intensity if you select the resistance correctly, as the final 10-second lowering will be challenging.

Katie Fellows Smith

Age 60, Height 5' 4¾"

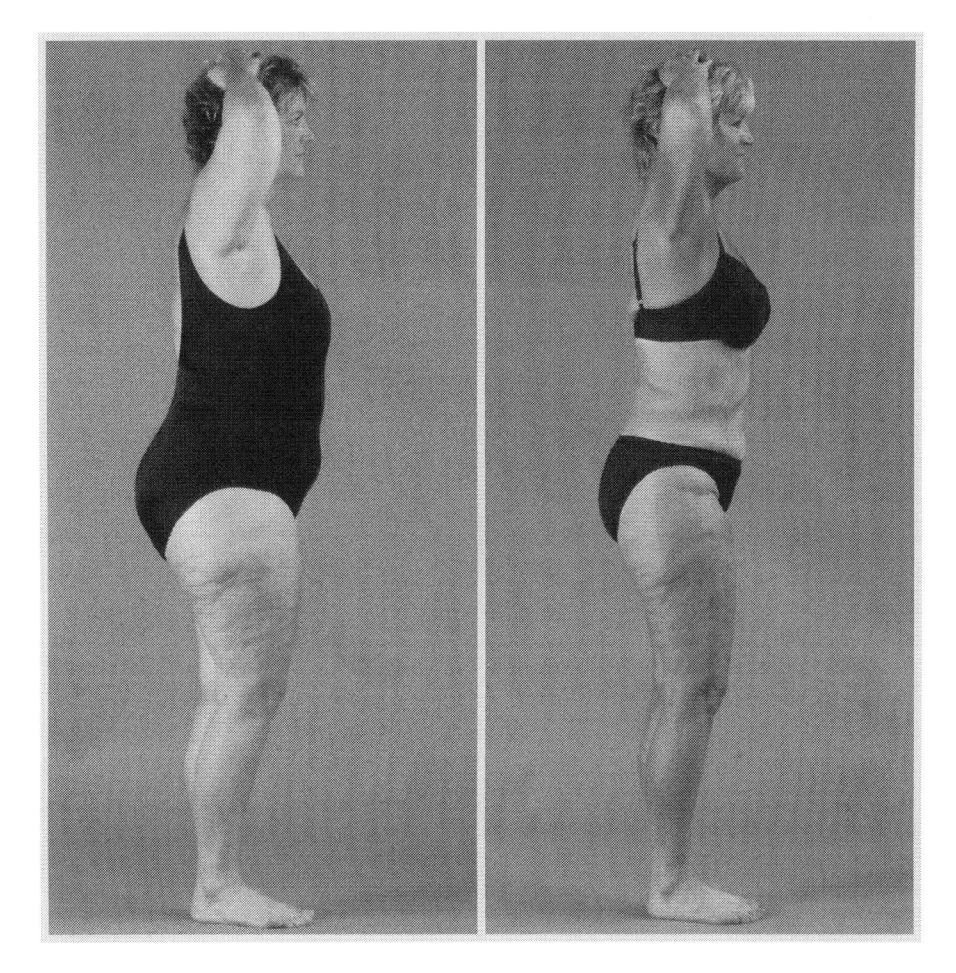

207.6 pounds   **152.1** pounds

After 18 weeks
62.75 pounds of fat loss,
9.125 inches off waist, **12** inches off thighs
7.23 pounds of muscle gain

"For twenty-seven years, I weighed over 200 pounds. I had almost given up hope of ever returning to a somewhat normal body weight. Then, I met Ellington Darden and he got me involved in his program. His 10-10-10 training was a miracle. Now look at me."

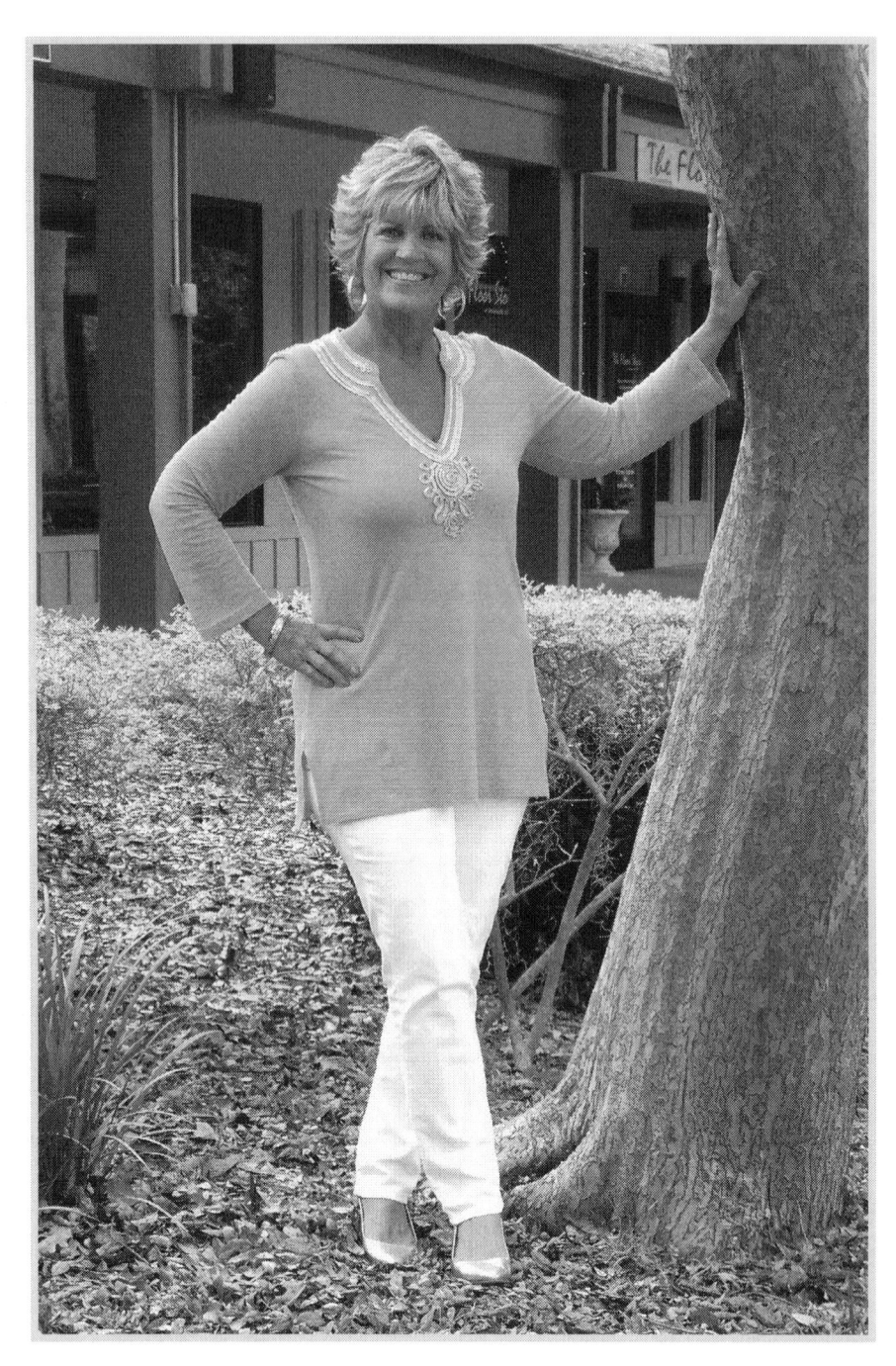

After losing almost 63 pounds of fat, Katie Smith said: "I feel full of life, flexible, and strong. Dr. Darden's 10-10-10 method makes it easy for me to train myself, and my strength is still increasing."

With 10-10-10, you get 30 to 40 seconds of the repetitions devoted to the negative in a set that lasts 50 seconds. And the entire set is controlled by the trainee. One set per exercise is the standard requirement.

Furthermore, 10-10-10 is adaptable to almost all dumbbell, barbell, and machine exercises.

LLS and the Negative Awakening

The acronym **LLS** stands for **Living Longer Stronger**, but it also works well for **Lift & Lower-Slower** strength training.

Lift & Lower-Slower training has been a popular, though unnamed, concept that I've adapted, revised, and written about for fifty years. Lift & Lower-Slower relates to multiple ways of accentuating the lowering or negative phase of strength training exercise.

Lift & Lower-Slower and **10-10-10** are now new parts of the Negative Awakening.

10-10-10 Review

Specific exercises are described in chapters 9 and 10. Before you start, let's review how the 10-10-10 method works regardless of the exercise.

Starting with a moderate amount of resistance for the selected exercise:

- Assume the appropriate starting position (see chapters 9 and 10, and read carefully).
- Lift the resistance smoothly to the top position.
- First negative rep: Lower under control for 10 seconds.
- Reps 1-9: Lift for 1 second, lower for 2 seconds.
- Rep 10: Lift for 1 second and hold steady at the top.
- Finish negative: Lower 10th rep under control in 10 seconds.

To review, there's a 10-second negative, then 10 normal reps with a hold at the top on the 10th, followed by a final 10-second negative . . . hence the name **10-10-10**.

Phase:	First **10**-Second Negative	**10** Normal Reps	Final **10**-Second Negative
Action:	(after the initial lift) Lower in a slow and controlled manner.	Reps 1–9: Lift for 1 second, lower for 2 seconds. Rep 10: Lift for 1 second and hold.	Lower the weight in a controlled manner.
Time to perform:	10 seconds	30 seconds total	10 seconds
Provides:	Intense focus on the involved muscles.	Inroad in a regular manner.	Deep isolation of the involved muscles for maximum stimulation.

Each 10-10-10 exercise takes approximately 50 seconds to complete.

When you can do the finish negative smoothly for a full 10 seconds, increase the resistance by 3 to 5 percent at your next workout.

Understand that once you get the hang of 10-10-10, your progression will not always be the ideal 10-10-10. Sometimes you will not be able to perform all 10 reps, and the finish negative may be too fast. For example, you might need to record an exercise as 10-9-7, 10-8-6, or even 10-11-10 if you were particularly strong on the exercise and did 11 regular reps instead of 10. The goal of 10-10-10 is simply an achievement that changes slightly during each workout. Do your best on each exercise.

Please practice the above instructions for the Darden 10-10-10 Method. It will prepare you for success in following the specific instructions for each exercise in chapters 9 and 10.

Remember, 10-10-10 emphasizes the negative or lowering phase of an exercise. Why? Because science shows that the lowering is the most productive part of the movement. Many trainees have neglected the lowering in the past and continue to make this mistake in the present. Don't be one of them.

You are about to experience Lift & Lower-Slower strength training and the Negative Awakening.

Still Living Longer 8 Stronger

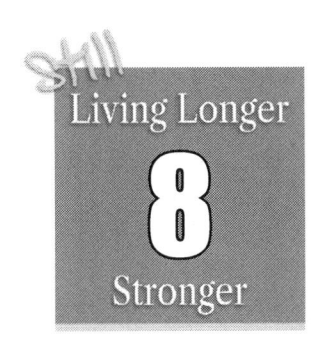

List of the Best 10-10-10 Exercises

I have more than sixty-five years of strength training experience, so I've seen it all and tried it all. Here's my list of recommended single-joint exercises and recommended multiple-joint exercises. Each exercise adapts well to the 10-10-10 style.

Best Single-Joint Exercises

- Leg extension on machine
- Leg curl on machine
- One-legged calf raise
- Standing calf raise on machine
- Biceps curl with barbell
- Hammer curl with dumbbells
- Triceps extension with one dumbbell
- Shoulder shrug with barbell
- Abdominal crunch machine

Best Multiple-Joint Exercises

- Squat with dumbbells
- Squat with barbell

Leg press on machine

Pulldown on lat machine

Overhead press with barbell

Bench press with barbell

Bent-over rowing with barbell

The above exercises require basic barbell and dumbbell bars, collars, and approximately 250 pounds of weight plates. If you are a member of a gym or fitness center, then you'll probably have access to various listed machines, such as the leg extension and leg curl. If doing these exercises at home, you can replace the barbell or dumbbells with items that have handles, such as paint cans, a laundry basket, bottles of laundry detergent, cases of water, a teapot with water, etc.

Each of the exercises will be described in the next two chapters.

Why Do 10-10-10 Reps Work?

The 10-10-10 method of strength training emphasizes the negative or lowering phase of each exercise. But, in simple terms, why do negative-emphasized reps cause your body to respond with greater strength?

Dr. Tim Olds, a Professor at the University of South Australia, has this answer:

"The involved muscle fibers are lengthening, but they are trying to contract at the same time as they are being pulled apart. This causes damage, and it's that, and the repair of it, which accounts for the benefits from eccentric training."

In other words, the lengthening muscles while striving to contract are elongated with controlled force. This results in the breaking of muscle fiber bonds, causing slight tearing, then soreness, and finally overcompensation. Combined with proper sleep, the overall effect is greater muscular size and strength.

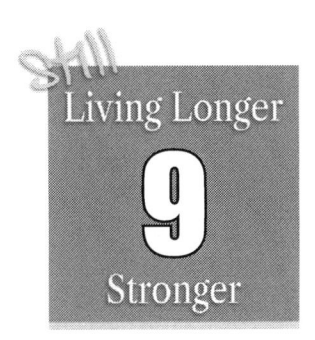

Single-Joint Exercises

There are nine single-joint exercises in this chapter. I chose them because, in my sixty-five years of strength training experience, I have found them to be effective, and because they are well suited to the 10-10-10 method.

In this chapter, I will teach you exactly how to apply the 10-10-10 method for each exercise. The steps are outlined under the following headings:

Preparation: Equipment required and starting position

First Negative: A description of the lowering phase of the movement

Regular Reps: An explanation of how to do the normal positive-negative reps

Finish Negative: A description of the final negative part of the exercise and how to make it more effective

Tips: Details to improve the results

Leg Extension Machine

Muscles worked: Quadriceps

Preparation

- Have a watch or a big clock with a second hand in plain sight, or have a spotter help with the counting. You can find a clock with a second hand online at: https://www.online-stopwatch.com/clocks/.

- Sit in the machine and place your feet and ankles behind the bottom roller pad.
- Align your knee joints with the axis of rotation of the movement arm.
- Fasten the seat belt, if one is provided, across your hips securely to keep your buttocks from rising.
- Lean back and stabilize your upper body by grasping the handles or the sides of the machine. With your spotter's assistance, smoothly lift the movement arm to the top position and pause.

First Negative

- Begin the lowering process. Move smoothly and slowly, about 1 inch per second.
- Try to be halfway down at 5 seconds and three-quarters down at 7 seconds.
- Keep your focus.
- Be at the bottom at 10 seconds, then turn the movement around smoothly and get ready for some regular reps.

Regular Reps

- Straighten your legs smoothly in 1 second.
- Pause briefly and lower the resistance in 2 seconds.
- Continue for 10 repetitions.
- Lean back, not forward, as your legs straighten.
- Hold the 10th rep at the top and stabilize your body for the finish negative.

Finish Negative

- Lower the weight smoothly by bending your legs slowly, about 1 inch per second.
- Be halfway down at 5 seconds and three-quarters down at 7 seconds.
- Relax your face and emphasize your breathing out.
- Fight the last few seconds and set the weight down at 10 seconds.
- Be careful as you exit the machine.

> ### Tips
>
> - Keep your feet straight ahead of you and in a neutral, relaxed position during all phases of the leg extension. Do not extend your toes or flex them.
> - Do not move your head forward or side to side.
> - Practice smooth turnarounds at both ends of the exercise.

Leg Curl Machine

Muscles worked: Hamstrings

Preparation

- Have a watch with a second hand in plain sight, or get a spotter to help with the initial lifting and counting.
- There are several versions of the leg curl machine, including prone, seated, and kneeling. This exercise uses the prone type, which is the most popular version.
- Lie face down on the leg curl machine with your knees on the pad edge closest to the movement arm.
- Hook your heels and ankles under the roller pad.
- Make sure your knee joints are in line with the axis of rotation of the movement arm.
- Grasp the handles on the edge of the machine bench to steady your upper body.
- Get the movement arm to the contracted position smoothly, either by yourself or with a spotter's assistance.

First Negative

- Hold the contracted position briefly and begin the negative.
- Lower slowly, about 1 inch per second.
- Try to be halfway down at 5 seconds and three-quarters down at 7 seconds.

- Touch the bottom at 10 seconds but do not rest. Turn the resistance around smoothly and start the regular-speed reps.

Regular Reps

- Lift the movement arm smoothly in 1 second to the top position and lower it in 2 seconds to the bottom.
- Do 10 repetitions, in good form.
- Hold the 10th repetition at the top for 1 second. Stabilize your body for the finish negative.

Finish Negative

- Ease out of the top position slowly.
- Lower smoothly and slowly, about 1 inch per second. Be at the halfway-down mark at 5 seconds.
- Keep your face relaxed, stay focused, and pass the three-quarters down mark at 7 seconds.
- Resist steadily and reach the bottom at 10 seconds.
- Relax your legs, scoot backwards, stand, and exit the machine.

Tips

- During both the negative and positive phases of the leg curl, flex your ankles so your toes are pointed toward your knees. This flexion of the ankle, called dorsiflexion, stretches your calves and allows for a greater range of motion of the hamstrings.
- Keep your chin forward during the exercise, as opposed to turning your face to either side.

One-Legged Calf Raise

Muscles worked: Gastrocnemius and soleus

Preparation

- Have a watch with a second hand in plain sight, or get a spotter to help with the initial lifting and counting.
- Find a step that has a secure ledge to stand on and a handrail to use for balance. The bottom step of a staircase works well.
- Wear rubber-soled shoes with treads on the bottom for better gripping with the soles of your feet.
- Stand on the step with both feet.
- Lift one foot and hold it behind your knee. Your entire body weight is now on the other foot.
- Raise the heel of the down foot so all your weight is on the ball of the foot. You'll now have your entire body weight on one foot, so you will have plenty of resistance with your body weight for several months.
- Contract the calf muscle of the down leg intensely and stabilize your body by holding onto the handrail lightly.

First Negative

- Lower your heel slowly, about ½ inch per second.
- Try to be halfway down at 5 seconds and all the way down at 10 seconds.
- Stretch at the bottom for 1 second and begin the positive/negative regular reps.

Regular Reps

- Raise your heel in 1 second to the contracted position and pause briefly.
- Do the negative phase in 2 seconds and stretch.
- Continue to perform the one-legged calf raise for 10 reps, in good form.
- Hold the 10th rep at the top and ready yourself for the finish negative.

Finish Negative

- Lower your heel very slowly, ½ inch per second.
- Be halfway down at 5 seconds. Keep your knee locked. Do not bend it.
- Do a deep stretch for one second at the 10-second mark.
- Step down from the ledge gently, one foot at a time, and relax.
- Switch legs and perform the one-legged calf raise for your other leg.

Tips

- It is especially important to move slowly and pause briefly at each turnaround.
- Pay attention to your balance and make sure you are standing on a stable step.

Calf Raise Machine

Muscles worked: Gastrocnemius and soleus

Preparation

- Have a watch with a second hand in plain sight, or get a spotter to help with the initial lifting and counting.
- There are various types of calf raise machines. The one described here is the standing version, with a thick ledge at the bottom to stand on.
- Wear rubber-soled shoes with treads on the bottom for better gripping with the soles of your feet.
- Adjust the shoulder pads for your height, if necessary, and place the balls of both feet on the ledge at the bottom.
- Stand and lift the resistance.
- Raise your heels, which contracts your calf muscles, and keep your knees stiff.
- Get as high as you can on your tiptoes and pause briefly.

First Negative

- Lower your heels very slowly, about ½ inch per second.
- Try to be halfway down at 5 seconds and three-quarters down at 7 seconds.
- Reach the bottom at 10 seconds, stretch briefly below the ledge, and begin the positive/negative regular reps.

Regular Reps

- Raise your heels in 1 second to the top and pause briefly.
- Do the negative phase in 2 seconds, then pause briefly and stretch.
- Continue to perform the calf raise for 10 reps, in good form.
- Hold the 10th rep at the top for 1 second and ready yourself for the finish negative.

Finish Negative

- Lower your heels very slowly, about ½ inch per second.
- Be halfway down at 5 seconds. Keep your knees locked. Do not bend them.
- Do a deep stretch at the 10-second mark.
- Step down from the ledge gently, one foot at a time, and relax.

Tips

- Keep your knees straight during the movement, especially the bottom-stretch phases.
- If you do the repetitions smoothly and slowly, you'll get a deep burn in your posterior calf muscles—and probably some calf soreness over the next several days. Stretch your calves gently for relief.

Biceps Curl with Barbell

Muscles worked: Biceps of upper arms

Preparation

- Have a watch or big clock with a second hand in plain sight, or have a spotter help with the counting.
- Grip the barbell underhand, with your hands shoulder-width apart.
- Stand with the barbell, then curl the weight smoothly to your shoulders.
- Anchor the elbows firmly against your sides in preparation for the first negative.

First Negative

- Lower the weight smoothly and slowly, about an inch per second. Keep your elbows anchored against your sides; do not move them backward.
- Reach the halfway-down position at 5 seconds.
- Keep your torso erect as you near the bottom at 10 seconds.
- Get ready to begin the faster-speed, positive/negative repetitions.

Normal Reps

- Curl the weight to your shoulders in approximately 1 second, then lower it smoothly in about 2 seconds. (That's a one-second positive and a 2-second negative.)
- Continue for 10 repetitions without resting in between, moving steadily and making the bottom and top turnarounds in a controlled manner.
- Stop at the top of the 10th repetition and ready yourself for the finish negative.

Finish Negative

- Lower the weight smoothly and slowly, about 1 inch per second.
- Be halfway down at 5 seconds, near the bottom at 7 seconds, and all the way down at 10 seconds.
- Place the barbell on the floor and relax.

> **Tips**
>
> - Maximize your biceps stimulation by minimizing your body sway backward and forward.
> - Do not lean forward excessively or lean backward. Do not move your upper arms. Do not move your head.
> - Move only your hands, your forearms, and the barbell.

Hammer Curl with Dumbbells

Muscles worked: Brachialis, biceps, and brachioradialis

Preparation

- Have a watch or big clock with a second hand in plain sight, or have a spotter help with the counting.
- Grasp a dumbbell in each hand and stand with your feet shoulder-width apart.
- Turn the dumbbells so your palms are facing your torso, like the way you'd hold and use a hammer.
- Smoothly curl the dumbbells to your shoulders.
- Anchor your elbows firmly against your sides and begin the first negative.

First Negative

Without leaning, moving your elbows away from your sides, or rotating your forearms:

- Lower the dumbbell together slowly, about 1 inch per second.
- Reach the halfway-down position at 5 seconds.
- Reach the bottom at 10 seconds.
- Get ready to begin the faster-speed, positive/negative repetitions.

Normal Reps

- Curl the dumbbells to your shoulders hammer-style in approximately 1 second, then lower it in 2 seconds (that's a 1-second positive and a 2-second negative).
- Continue for 10 repetitions without resting in between, moving steadily and making the bottom and top turnarounds in a controlled manner.
- Stop at the top of the 10th repetition and ready yourself for the finish negative.

Finish Negative

- Lower the dumbbells smoothly and slowly using your brachialis and biceps, about 1 inch per second.
- Be halfway down at 5 seconds, near the bottom at 7 seconds, and all the way down at 10 seconds.
- Place the dumbbells on the floor and relax.

Tips

- Maximize your brachialis and biceps stimulation by minimizing your body sway.
- Do not lean forward excessively or lean backward. Do not move your upper arms. Do not move your head.
- Move only your hands, your forearms, and the dumbbells.

Triceps Extension with One Dumbbell

Muscles worked: Triceps

Preparation

- Have a watch or a big clock with a second hand in plain sight, or have a spotter help with counting.
- Sit on a bench. Grasp the shaft of a dumbbell with both hands and hold it out in front of you.

- Pull your elbows in so that your arms are more or less straight.
- Keeping your arms straight, raise the dumbbell up until it is above your head and your elbows are close to your ears. (Keep your elbows there throughout the exercise.)

First Negative

Keeping your elbows close to your ears, moving only your forearms and hands:

- Bend your elbows slowly to lower the dumbbell, moving about an inch per second.
- Reach the halfway-down position at 5 seconds, and the bottom position (the dumbbell behind your neck) at 10 seconds.
- Turn the resistance around and begin the regular positive/negative reps.

Regular Reps

- Extend the dumbbell smoothly overhead in 1 second and immediately lower it in 2 seconds.
- Do 10 repetitions in good form.
- Stop at the top of the 10th repetition and begin the finish negative.

Finish Negative

- Repeat the procedure for the first negative, reaching the halfway point at 5 seconds and the bottom at 10 seconds.
- Focus and keep good form. Relax your face and breathe.
- Bend forward slightly at the waist, lift the dumbbell over one shoulder with both hands and place it on the floor. Or have the spotter grasp the dumbbell from behind your neck.

Tips

- Move in and out of the bottom position very carefully, with no jerks, to avoid strains to the triceps.

Shoulder Shrug with Barbell

Muscles worked: Trapezius

Preparation

- Have a watch or big clock with a second hand in plain sight, or have a spotter help with the counting.
- This is a short-range movement, so you need to perform the details with precision.
- Take an overhand grip on a barbell. Your hands should be slightly wider apart than your shoulders.
- Stand erect to lift the barbell. The bar should now be touching your thighs.
- Using only your shoulders, as when shrugging, lift the barbell smoothly as high as possible.
- Pause no more than two seconds as you ready yourself for the negative.

First Negative

- Lean forward slightly and bend your knees a little. Stay this way through all phases.
- Begin reversing the shrug to lower the barbell slowly, ½ inch per second.
- Be halfway down at 5 seconds and three-quarters down at 7 seconds.
- Sag your shoulders forward and downward as far as comfortably possible at 10 seconds.
- Then proceed directly into the regular reps with no pause.

Regular Reps

- Gripping the bar firmly, shrug your shoulders up in 1 second and down in 2 seconds, for 10 reps.
- Stop at the top of the 10th rep to be ready for the finish negative.

Finish Negative

- Reverse the shrug slowly to lower the barbell.
- Be halfway down at 5 seconds and all the way down at 10 seconds.

- Pause briefly in the down position.
- Place the barbell on the floor, stand, and relax.

Tips

- Practice keeping your arms straight and mostly relaxed when shrugging. If you bend your arms, your biceps will be brought into action.
- Keep a slight arch in your back throughout the movement.

Abdominal Crunch Machine

Muscles worked: Rectus abdominis and external obliques

Preparation

- Have a watch or big clock with a second hand in plain sight, or have a spotter to help with counting.
- Many different types of abdominal machines are manufactured today. I like the ones that put the user in an upright, seated position, with a pivot point at the midsection and a movement arm slightly above the shoulders.
- Adjust the seat height so your navel, when you are seated, is level with the machine's pivot point.
- Fasten the seat belt across your hips, then cross your ankles.
- Place your elbows on the pads and grasp the handles lightly.
- Get to the contracted position smoothly by pulling with your elbows and ready yourself for the first negative.

First Negative

Breathing freely and keeping your face relaxed:

- Return the movement arm to the top position slowly, about ½ inch per second, by releasing your abdominal muscles.

- Be halfway back at 5 seconds and three-quarters back at 7 seconds.
- Be ready to turn around the movement at the stretched, top position to start regular reps.

Regular Reps

- Pull with your elbows and begin shortening the distance between your lower ribs and pelvis. Be sure and breathe.
- Keeping the movement continuous, do a 1-second positive followed by a 2-second negative.
- Do 10 reps.
- Pause briefly in the contracted position of the 10th rep.
- Turn around the movement and start the finish negative.

Finish Negative

- Keep your back rounded as you slowly release or lengthen your abdominal muscles. Open your eyes, and focus on the count.
- Moving smoothly and slowly, about ½ inch per second, be halfway back at 5 seconds and three-quarters back at 7 seconds.
- Arch your back slightly near the top position and allow the weight stack to touch at the count of 10 seconds.
- Relax and exit the machine.

Tips

- Keep your shoulders against the seat back throughout the movement. Do not push your chin forward at the start of the positive.
- Do not try to do a sit-up on this machine.
- Try to bring your ribcage closer to your pelvic girdle.
- Do not pull excessively with your arms.
- Pull with your midsection muscles.

Single-Joint Exercises 75

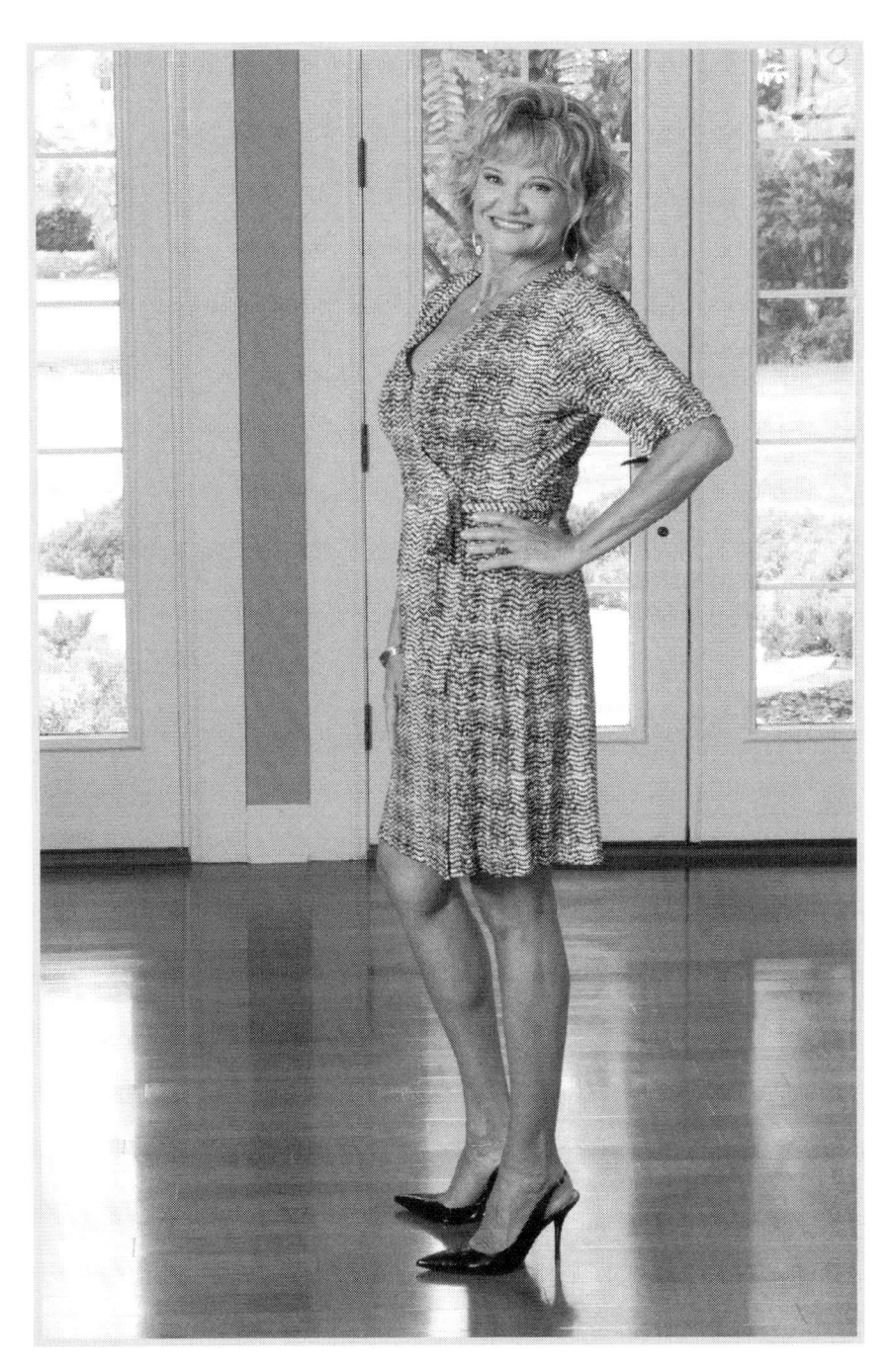

Mary Dees, age 61, lost 17.75 pounds of fat and gained 2.9 pounds of muscle. "Dr. D opened my eyes to having a plan, learning to stick with it, and understanding how to say NO!"

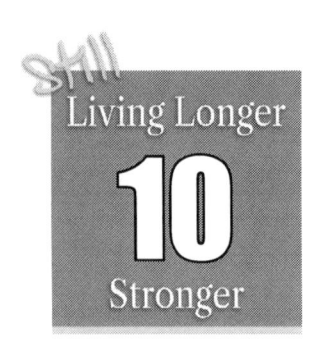

Multiple-Joint Exercises

A multiple-joint exercise involves two or more joints. There are seven multiple-joint exercises in this chapter. I chose them for the SLLS program because of their long range of movement.

The exercises in this chapter will be described in the same manner as those in the previous chapter.

Squat with Dumbbells

Muscles worked: Gluteus maximus, quadriceps, hamstrings, and erector spinae

Preparation

- Have a watch or big clock with a second hand in plain sight, or have a spotter help with the counting.
- Grasp a dumbbell in each hand and stand. The dumbbells should be hanging down by the outside of your thighs.
- Place your feet a little farther than shoulder width apart, with your toes angled out slightly.
- Keep your upper-body muscles rigid, chest out, and torso upright.

First Negative

For this exercise, think of your arms as hangers, with the dumbbells at the ends. You will push your hips and butt back as if you were going to close a door behind you with your butt. Keep your heels on the floor and a slight arch in your lower back throughout the exercise.

- Start bending your knees slightly, moving about 1 inch per second.
- Continue to descend, reaching the half-squat position at the 5-second mark and a three-quarters squat at 7 seconds.
- Go as low as you can without lifting your heels. Be at your lowest level at 10 seconds. The dumbbells should almost touch the floor.
- Push down through your heels, not your toes, and get ready to do the regular reps.

Regular Reps

Keeping your chest high and your breathing regular:

- Begin immediately doing the 10 faster reps.
- Perform these smoothly, taking 1 second on the positive and 2 seconds on the negative.
- Push yourself to do 10 repetitions. Remember, the regular repetitions may vary between 8 and 12. The idea is to do as many as you can, in good form.
- Get ready for the finish negative.

Finish Negative

Breathing, focusing on the count, and keeping your torso rigid:

- Repeat the slow lowering.
- Be halfway down at 5 seconds. The hardest part is from halfway down to the bottom.
- Place the dumbbells on the floor at 10 seconds. Stand and relax your thighs.

Tips

- Note that your shape and flexibility can affect how deeply you can squat with the dumbbells. Some people have difficulty squatting below a level where the tops of their thighs are parallel to the floor. Others can almost touch their buttocks to their heels.
- If your ankles are tight and you tend to lift your heels at the bottom of the squat, try placing a 1-inch-thick board under your heels for stability.

Squat With Barbell

Muscles worked: Gluteus maximus, quadriceps, hamstrings, and erector spinae

Preparation

- Have a watch or big clock with a second hand in plain sight, or have a spotter help with the counting.
- Place a barbell inside a power rack in the top position on the hooks.
- Take two horizontal restraint bars and place them appropriately in the lowest deep-squat position of your range of motion. These bars protect you from going too low, losing your balance, and possibly injuring yourself.
- Load the barbell with the appropriate amount of resistance.
- Position the bar behind your neck across your trapezius muscles and hold the bar in place with your hands. If the bar cuts into your skin, pad it lightly by wrapping a towel around the knurl.
- Straighten your knees to lift the bar from the hooks, then move back one step.
- Place your feet shoulder-width apart, toes angled slightly outward. Keep your upper body muscles rigid and your torso upright during this exercise.

First Negative

- Bend your hips and knees slowly, about 1 inch per second.
- Descend gradually, reaching the half-squat position by 5 seconds.
- Squat a little farther to three-quarters level.
- Reach the bottom position, in which your hamstrings firmly meet your calves, by 10 seconds.
- Make the turnaround gradually from negative to positive.

Regular Reps

- Perform 10 barbell squats smoothly at a speed of 1 second for the positive and 2 seconds for the negative.
- Push yourself and complete 10 repetitions. The regular repetitions may vary between 8 and 12. The idea is to do as many as you can, in good form.

- Get ready, after your last rep, for the finish negative.

Finish Negative

Keeping your focus, and continuing to breathe:

- Bend your hips and knees smoothly and slowly.
- Hit the halfway-down mark at 5 seconds and the three-quarters mark at 7 seconds.
- Hold the resistance off the bottom restraint bars, in the deep-squat position, for a final second or two.
- Transfer the barbell to the bottom restraint bars. Sit down on the floor, or move away from the power rack carefully, and relax.

> **Tips**
>
> - Do not allow your torso to bend forward on the positive reps of the squat. Doing so takes some of the force off your thighs and places it on your lower back, which can be dangerous.
> - As a safety measure, it's also a good idea to use at least one spotter, preferably two, during the barbell squat.

Leg Press Machine

Muscles worked: Gluteals, quadriceps, and hamstrings

Preparation

- Have a watch or big clock with a second hand in plain sight, or get a spotter to help with the initial lifting and counting.
- There are many versions of the leg press machine. This exercise is for the kind with a diagonal movement arm, or footboard.
- Sit in the machine with your back against the angled pad and your buttocks on the seat bottom.
- Place your feet on the footboard with your heels shoulder-width apart and your toes pointed slightly outward.

- Straighten your legs and release the stop bars of the machine (be sure to lock these stop bars at the end of your set to secure the footboard).
- Grasp the handles beside the seat, or the edge of the seat, during the exercise.

First Negative

- Lower the footboard slowly by bending your hips and knees.
- Try to be halfway down at 5 seconds and three-quarters down at 7 seconds.
- Turn the resistance around smoothly at 10 seconds. Do not stop and rest at the bottom. Barely touch, then immediately start the regular reps.

Regular Reps

- Leg-press the footboard and weight smoothly to the top in 1 second and return it to the bottom in 2 seconds.
- Make sure the turnarounds at the bottom and top are carefully done. Do not bounce the weight at any time.
- Continue for 10 reps.
- Stop the 10th repetition at the top in preparation for a slow finish negative.

Finish Negative

Focus intensely, and remember: You have more strength in the negative than the positive. You're still strong enough to do a final 10-second negative. Doing so successfully is the most important of these phases.

Keeping your face relaxed, and continuing to breathe freely:

- Lower the footboard very slowly, about 1 inch per second.
- Be at the halfway-down position at 5 seconds and three-quarters down at 7 seconds. The hardest portion is the last several seconds.
- Don't set the footboard on the stops until 10 seconds are completed.
- Have your spotter help you out of the machine or assist you in pressing the resistance back to the top position.

> **Tips**
>
> - The leg press is a very demanding exercise.
> - Work diligently on keeping your movement slow and continuous. Practice keeping your face and neck relaxed.

Pulldown on Lat Machine

Muscles worked: Biceps and latissimus dorsi

Preparation

- Have a watch or a big clock with a second hand in plain sight, or have a spotter help with counting.
- Grasp the pulldown bar on a lat machine with an underhand, shoulder-width grip, then sit down.
- Stabilize your lower body properly by using your legs.
- Pull the bar down to your chest smoothly, which lifts the resistance, and ready yourself for the negative.

First Negative

- Pause briefly with the bar touching your upper chest. Your elbows should be down and back and held steady.
- Begin unbending your arms and lowering the resistance slowly, about 1 inch per second.
- Be halfway down at 5 seconds and three-quarters down at 7 seconds.
- Stretch your arms at the top and turn around the bar at 10 seconds.

Regular Reps

- Pull the bar smoothly to your chest in 1 second.
- Lower the bar to the bottom in 2 seconds.
- Continue to lift and lower for 10 repetitions.
- Pause briefly at the bottom of the 10th repetition and turn around the movement for the finish negative.

Finish Negative

- Unbend your elbows and lower the resistance slowly, about 1 inch per second.
- Be halfway down at 5 seconds and three-quarters down at 7 seconds.
- Stay in control and breathe freely.
- Stretch your arms and upper back at 10 seconds.
- Allow the resistance to bottom out on the weight stack, then stand and exit the machine.

Tips

- Keep your torso upright during the negative phases.
- Minimize body sway and practice strict form.

Overhead Press with Barbell

Muscles worked: Deltoids and triceps

Even with a 30-pound barbell, this is a tough, challenging exercise. Be careful.

Preparation

- Have a watch or a big clock with a second hand in plain view, or have a spotter help with counting.
- Place a barbell on mid-chest-high hooks in a power rack.
- Load the bar with an appropriate amount of weight.
- Grasp the barbell with an overhand grip and position your hands slightly wider than your shoulders.
- Unhook and lift the barbell, mostly with your legs, and step back with it on your shoulders. Make sure your feet and legs are in a stable position.
- Bend your knees slightly and push-press the barbell overhead. With your elbows completely straight, the barbell should be

directly above your shoulders. Ready yourself for the negative phase, as you'll be lowering the bar to your shoulders.

First Negative

- Lower the barbell slowly, about 1 inch per second.
- Be halfway down at 5 seconds and three-quarters down at 7 seconds.
- Focus on your breathing.
- Touch your upper chest at 10 seconds and turn around the movement.

Regular Reps

- Begin your regular-speed barbell presses smoothly, taking 1 second for the positive and 2 seconds for the negative.
- Try to complete 10 repetitions.
- Stop at the top of the 10th repetition and ready yourself for the finish negative.

Finish Negative

- Guide the barbell down slowly, about an inch per second.
- Move past the halfway point at 5 seconds and past the three-quarters point at 7 seconds.
- Try to control the movement by breathing out at a rapid rate.
- Touch your upper chest at 10 seconds.
- Move back carefully to the power rack and place the bar securely on the hooks.
- Exit the power rack and relax.

Tips

- Keep your lower back naturally arched during the movements.
- It may take you several practice sessions to learn the mechanics of the negative-accentuated overhead press.
- This is an excellent exercise for your shoulders and arms, although it can be somewhat challenging for both women and men.

Chest Press Machine

Muscles worked: Pectoralis major, deltoid, and triceps

Preparation

- Have a watch or a big clock with a second hand in plain sight, or have a spotter help with counting.
- Adjust the seat bottom on the chest machine so your hands can comfortably grasp the bottom handles of the movement arm.
- Sit tall and grasp the handles. Keep your shoulder blades together throughout the movement.
- Straighten your elbows and move the weight stack smoothly to the top position, or get assistance from your spotter.

First Negative

- Lower the resistance slowly, about 1 inch per second.
- Reach the halfway-down level at 5 seconds and the three-quarters down point at 7 seconds.
- Continue the controlled lowering and reach the bottom at 10 seconds.
- Turn the resistance around smoothly and begin the positive/negative regular-speed reps.

Regular Reps

- Move out of the bottom smoothly and press to the top without jerking.
- Do the negative a little slower than you did the positive.
- Repeat the movement for 10 reps.
- At the end of the 10th rep, prepare for a finish negative.

Finish Negative

Staying in control, keeping your face relaxed, and breathing freely:

- Fight the lowering, moving smoothly.
- Be halfway down at 5 seconds and completely down at 10 seconds.
- Ease off the movement gradually. Remove your hands from the handles and relax.

> **Tips**
>
> - Do not move your hips during the positive phase, nor arch your back excessively.
> - Do not move your feet during either the negative or positive movements. Keep them on the floor.

Bench Press with Barbell

Muscles worked: Pectoralis major, deltoids, and triceps

The first time you do this exercise using the 10-10-10 method, use only 60 percent of the weight you would normally use for 10 repetitions.

Preparation

- Have a watch or big clock with a second hand in plain sight, or have a spotter help with counting.
- Set up a barbell with appropriate resistance on the support racks of a flat bench.
- Lie on your back on the bench.
- Grasp the barbell with your hands positioned slightly farther apart than the width of your shoulders.
- Straighten your arms and bring the barbell to a supported position above your sternum.

First Negative

- Lower the barbell slowly, about 1 inch per second.
- Try to be halfway down at 5 seconds and three-quarters down at 7 seconds.
- Touch your sternum at 10 seconds, but do not rest.
- Make a smooth turnaround and get ready to begin the faster-speed positive/negative repetitions.

Regular Reps

- Press the barbell in approximately 1 second to full extension.
- Lower the bar smoothly in approximately 2 seconds.
- Make the bottom and top turnarounds under control and continue for 10 steady repetitions, without resting.
- Stop at the top of the 10th repetition and ready yourself for the finish negative.

Finish Negative

- Lower the bar in a slow, smooth, and controlled manner, about 1 inch per second.
- Be at the halfway-down point at 5 seconds.
- Fight the lowering. Don't let the resistance force the bar downward too fast.
- Reach the bottom at 10 seconds.
- Have the spotter quickly help you get the barbell back to the support racks at the top.
- Move off the bench and relax.

Tips

- This exercise takes some practice. Play it safe and use only 60 percent of what you'd normally handle for 10 repetitions during your first workout.
- Stabilize your starting position by squeezing your shoulder blades together and holding them that way throughout the exercise. Make sure the bar always remains directly above your elbows.
- Avoid using a wide grip on the bench press. Since the function of your pectoral muscles is to move your upper arms across your torso, spacing your hands wider than your shoulders shortens your range of motion. Rather than working more of your chest muscles, you're working less of them.
- Use a spotter on the barbell bench press.

Bent-Over Row with Barbell

Muscles worked: Latissimus dorsi and biceps

Preparation

- Have a watch or big clock with a second hand in plain sight, or have a spotter help with the counting.
- Set up a barbell with appropriate resistance on the floor.
- Place your feet close together under the bar.
- Bend over and grasp the barbell with an underhand grip. Your hands should be approximately 4 inches apart. Your torso should remain parallel to the floor.
- Keep a slight bend in your knees to reduce the stress on your lower back.
- Pull the barbell up your thighs and pause.

First Negative

- Lower the barbell slowly, about 1 inch per second.
- Be halfway down in 5 seconds and all the way down in 10 seconds.
- Stretch briefly at the bottom and ready yourself for the positive-negative reps.

Regular Reps

- Do your regular-speed reps smoothly, taking 1 second for the positive and 2 seconds for the negative.
- Pause at the top of the 10th rep and do the finish negative.

Finish Negative

- Lower the barbell slowly.
- Be halfway down at 5 seconds. Feel the movement intensely.
- Stretch in the bottom at the 10-second count.
- Place the barbell on the floor.

Tips

- Emphasize your latissimus dorsi more by rowing with an underhand grip. This places your biceps in a stronger position.
- Pause in the top position and try to pinch your shoulder blades together.

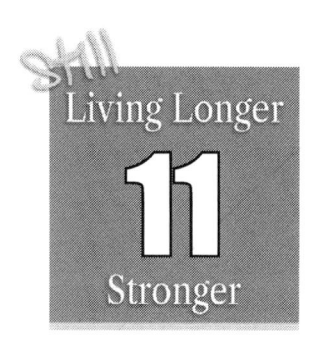

Proactive Eating

Proactive eating is a way of gaining control over your food consumption. When you understand the nutritional variables that affect your body composition, you can manipulate them for better health.

The Still Living Longer Stronger program involves proactive eating. This starts with having a working knowledge of your nutrient needs.

Recommended Dietary Allowance (RDA)

The RDAs are the levels of essential nutrients that are adequate to meet the known needs of all healthy individuals. These levels are established by the Committee on Dietary Allowances, part of the Food and Nutrition Board at the National Research Council.

RDA standards are revised every five to six years. Guidelines are listed according to sex, age, and weight for protein, eleven vitamins, and seven minerals.

It is important to understand that the RDAs are recommended daily averages. They are not requirements nor minimums, but they do include the differing needs of individuals. As a result, these allowances are several times higher than most people need. According to Dr. Fredrick Stare, founder of the Department of Nutrition at Harvard University's School of Public Health, "intakes equivalent to half of the RDAs are usually adequate."

Dr. Victor Herbert, a member of a past RDA committee, has noted that health hustlers often imply that individuals should consume more than the RDAs in case they have greater than average needs. This is not necessary; the RDAs are set high enough to encompass individual variations.

Food-Group Systems

Remember the four basic food groups? Generally, this fifty-year-old advice still makes a good foundation. The big difference in the system today is that the number of basic food groups is now six: fruit, vegetables, grains, protein foods, dairy products, and oils.

This new food plan, introduced by the US Department of Agriculture in 2020, designates fruits and vegetables as separate groups. Compared to the old system, it recommends more servings of fruits, vegetables, and grains and fewer of meat and dairy. Eating plans based on this system get most of their calories from carbohydrates and are limited in fats.

The emphasis in proactive eating is clearly on carbohydrates. At least 50 percent of your calories each day should come from carbohydrate-rich foods, with the rest from proteins, fats, and dairy.

The suggestions below are meant as a guide rather than a prescription. Skipping one group entirely for a day or so shouldn't be harmful if your overall eating plan is on track.

Guidelines for Healthy Eating

My Still Living Longer Stronger guidelines for proactive eating are based on my study of the standard recommendations of the US Department of Agriculture, the Surgeon General's Report, the American Heart Association, and the National Cancer Institute, plus my experience:

- Keep your total fat intake at 20 percent of your daily calories. Limit your intake of fat by selecting lean meats, poultry without skin, fish, and low-fat dairy products. In addition, cut back on vegetable oils, butter, and foods made with them (such as mayonnaise, salad dressings, and fried foods).

- Limit your intake of saturated fat to less than 10 percent of your fat calories. A diet high in saturated fat contributes to high blood cholesterol levels. The richest sources of saturated fat are animal products and tropical vegetable oils, such as coconut or palm oil.
- Decrease your cholesterol intake to 300 milligrams or less per day. Cholesterol is found only in animal products, such as meats, poultry, dairy products, and egg yolks.
- Consume a diet high in complex carbohydrates. Carbohydrates should contribute 50 percent or more of your total daily calories. To help meet this requirement, eat five or more servings daily of a combination of vegetables and fruits and six or more servings daily of whole grains or legumes. This will help you obtain the 20 to 30 grams of dietary fiber you need each day, as well as important vitamins and minerals.
- Maintain a moderate protein intake. Protein should make up about 20 percent of your total daily calories if you are trying to lose body fat. If you are trying to maintain your leanness, your protein can go down to 10 percent and your carbohydrates can move up to 70 percent. Choose low-fat sources of protein.
- Eat a variety of foods. Don't try to fill your nutrient requirements by consuming the same foods every day. Experiment with new and different foods—and read the labels carefully.
- Avoid too much sugar. Many foods that are high in sugar are also high in fat. Sugar also contributes to tooth decay.
- Lower your sodium intake to 2,400 milligrams per day. This is equal to the amount of sodium in a little more than a teaspoon of salt. Cut back on your use of the salt shaker and salt in cooking. Avoid salty prepackaged foods; check labels for salt and ingredients that contain sodium, such as condiments, pickles, and most cheeses.
- Emphasize an adequate calcium intake. Calcium is essential for strong bones and teeth. Get your calcium from dairy products or from substitutes such as almond milk, soy milk, and oat milk.
- Don't drink alcohol. Excess alcohol consumption can lead to a variety of health problems. And alcoholic beverages can add many calories to your diet without supplying other nutrients.
- Drink more water, especially if you are trying to lose fat.

The Well-Established Bottom Line

Many fitness-minded people believe that basic nutrition advice in the United States keeps changing—that the RDAs, food groups, and eating guidelines are always in a state of flux. But that is not the case.

Dr. Marion Nestle, professor emerita of nutrition at New York University, said in 2023 that recommendations have been remarkably consistent for the last seventy years. Yes, science has evolved, but the bottom-line dietary guidelines are stable: *Eat a variety of foods, in moderation, from the basic groups.*

That's still great advice you can use personally and pass on to your grandkids.

Roxanne Dybevick

Age 54, Height 5' 5"

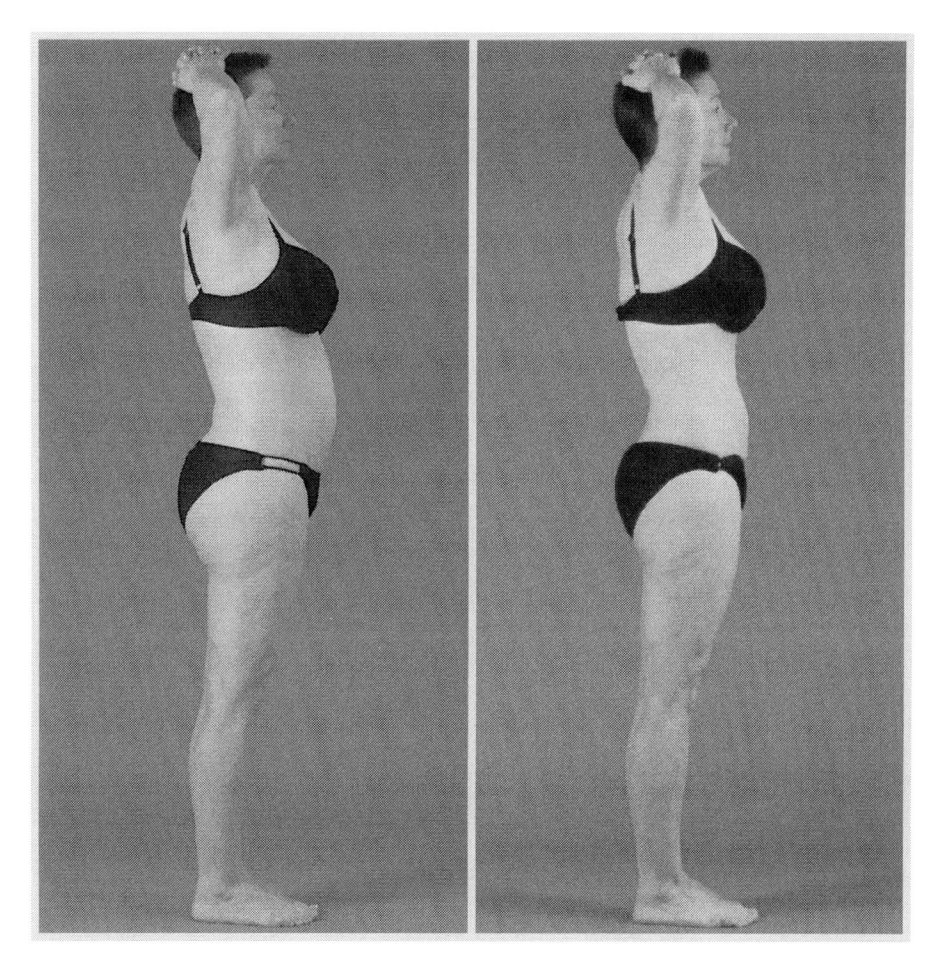

164 pounds   146.6 pounds

After 6 weeks
23.4 pounds of fat loss, **4.25** inches off waist
5.97 pounds of muscle gain

"We were presented this wonderful eating plan on paper:
This is exactly what you are going to eat each day.
It worked like a magic charm. It's like I now
have a second life, a second chance."

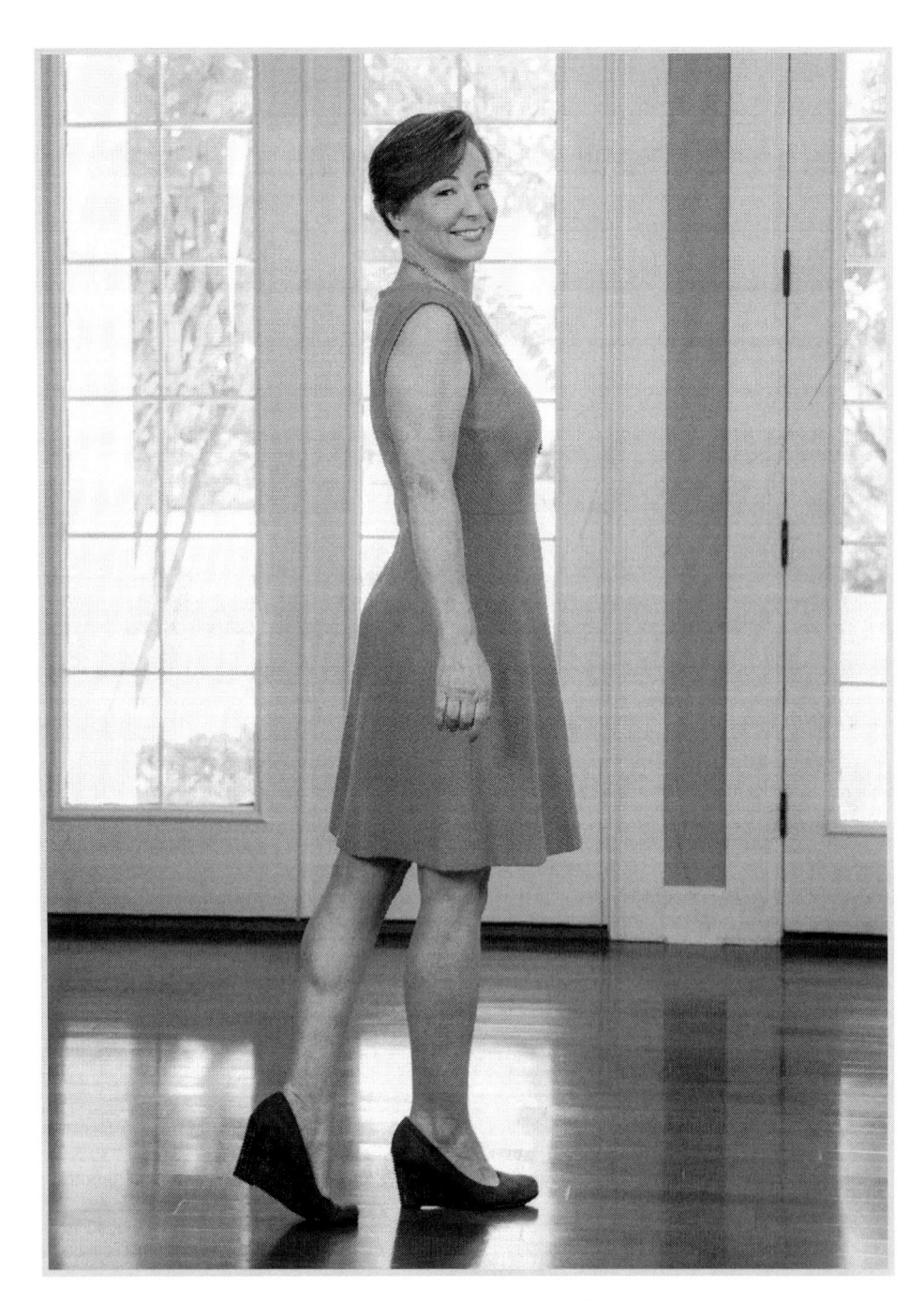

After losing 23 pounds of fat and building 6 pounds of muscle, Roxanne Dybevick noted: "I feel like an enthusiastic woman in her mid-twenties. I am excited now about my body, mind, and future."

Roxanne Shares

In her class of twenty-one women, Roxanne Dybevick finished first in pounds of fat lost. She kept a day-to-day journal of her experiences and thoughts as she progressed through the six-week course. The following excerpt is from Day 22, and it sheds some light on why many individuals over 75 years of age (me included) like to clean their plates when they eat and feel guilty afterward if they don't.

The Clean Plate Club and a Coyote

After addressing my demons directly for the past 22 days, I am more clearly seeing the family patterns that have dictated my behaviors that have in turn contributed to the layer of fat residing on my body. My mother, who lives near me in Gainesville, grew up during the era of the "CLEAN PLATE CLUB."

President Herbert Hoover in the early 1930s knew that many Americans had a strong sense of patriotism during World War I, trying to protect scarce food supplies and use supplies more efficiently. He used this to his advantage when he advertised the idea of the "Clean Plate" campaign.

In a previous entry I described how my mother was actually physically restrained, tied to the chair at the table, and asked to eat her meal. If not eaten completely, then that the plate was brought out night after night until it was eaten, every single morsel. My mother's treatment was an act of patriotism and a way her parents contributed to the success of the United States.

All this in a plate of food. I believe we are ALL members of the club, whether we know it or not.

Recently, my mother and I were driving around town running errands and I casually asked her what INTERESTING things happened to her at the dinner table growing up. I was expecting some stimulating historical family dinner conversation that might have happened around my grandparents' table. What my mother described was QUITE remarkable.

Mother described during the depression when people were out of jobs, they would come by the house and ask for work—to try and earn money for FOOD. This was a frequent occurrence. My mother's family was living in Lafayette, Indiana, in a large historic-type home. The type of home that could house a family of four, plus room for hired help.

My mother then mentioned a woman coming by the house and needing a place to live and my grandmother, having a big heart, agreeing she could live in the attic and work around the house for her keep. This woman then asked if her pet could come along and explained that it would be no trouble. Her pet turned out to be an emotional coyote.

My mother went on to detail the family sitting around the table eating a meal. The whole family attended grandma's dinners, with all the formality involved in being an army officer's wife. Grandpa at one end of the table and Grandma at the other end. The family circled around. The coyote living in the attic would bay, the crystal water glasses on the table vibrating to the soulful, mournful, wailing sound. Night after night after night.

The coyote, explained my mother, was actually trying to communicate with other coyotes. Except we were living in the middle of the city and there were no other coyotes in the area. What we had was a lonely, frustrated coyote. This continued for several months, and the family went on about their business of living and conversations were elevated to hear each other over the nonstop soulful howl. My mom had me laughing and thinking, laughing and thinking.

Analyzing everything, I now have a different opinion: I think the coyote, rather than being young and immature, was old and wise. Thus, through his howling, he was asking other coyotes to help my mother. To please take her away to the safety of the coyote den where they could eat when hungry and express themselves freely. Had the wise coyote been successful in contacting his pack, perhaps this story would have had a different ending.

Anyway, the point is today families are still members of the "Clean Plate Club." I believe it is time to disband the club. My mother, at 81 years old, still looks for the smallest plate in the house to eat on, as if the old club rules are still in effect.

Today is the halfway point in the program and I must admit, in just three short weeks, my attitude has completely changed. I find myself empowered as a woman, feeling like "I AM BACK." Yes, BACK in the game. The layer of fat was smothering my confidence and crushing my dreams. I had become literally someone I didn't recognize. I have lost 14 pounds. I have not cheated ONCE on the program and I am pleased by the results.

The BIGGEST change has not been my weight but my feelings about myself. I have adapted to the new way of living stronger. It is a commitment. A commitment to myself. To my health. And to my future.

I have eaten in the coyote den—and I have learned. I am wiser.

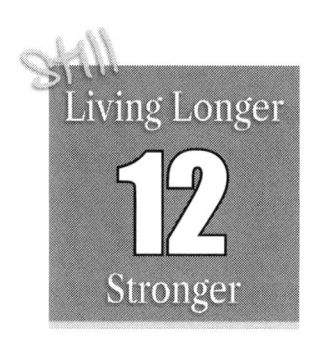

Nutrition Fallacies and Facts

From 1959 through 1969, I was a food faddist. I took thousands of dollars' worth of vitamin and mineral pills, protein tablets, and exotic powders such as desiccated liver, kelp, and brewer's yeast. At the same time, I avoided white bread, soft drinks, and processed meats. I was convinced that this eating program would help me become a superior athlete.

Where did I acquire these beliefs? Most of them came from physical fitness and health magazines. According to these publications, most recent champions had followed such a program. I never questioned these concepts until I entered graduate school at Florida State University. In fact, I kept trying to find new or more concentrated protein supplements to be certain that I was consuming more than 300 grams of protein per day—about four times as much as I needed.

Meeting Harold Schendel

During my first postgraduate year, I attended a seminar at which Dr. Harold E. Schendel spoke on the role of nutrition in physical fitness. Dr. Schendel was a professor of nutrition at Florida State and had spent four years in Africa and elsewhere directing research on problems of protein malnutrition. He had more than seventy published papers to his credit.

Dr. Schendel disagreed, to say the least, with most of my nutritional concepts. He did not believe my special eating habits were necessary, beneficial, or even safe. According to him, a fitness-minded person did not require large amounts of vitamins, proteins, or any special foods.

Over the next several months, Dr. Schendel and I had many friendly arguments concerning my practices and his scientific beliefs. Finally, he suggested that we collaborate on some research using me as a subject. *Great,* I thought. *Finally, I'll be able to prove to Dr. Schendel and other scientists that athletes like me really require massive amounts of essential nutrients.*

For two months, I kept precise records of my dietary intake, my energy expenditure, and how I felt. All my urine was collected and analyzed by a graduate research team in nutrition science.

Nutrient Overconsumption

The results of this study started me thinking in a different direction.

According to the RDAs, my protein need at that time was 77 grams per day. To my surprise, whenever I consumed more than that, the excess was excreted.

Worse than that, it was also determined that since I had been consuming massive doses of protein for many years, I had forced my liver and kidneys to grow excessively large to handle the influx of these proteins. An overly large liver and kidneys can cause several medical complications.

When I consumed more than the RDA of various vitamins and minerals, excess amounts of these substances were also excreted rather than being used by my body. Similar observations had been made by nutrition scientists since the 1930s, but it took a personal experience to undo the brainwashing I had undergone during my early years as an athlete.

The knowledge I gained while earning my PhD in exercise science, combined with more recently published nutritional studies, proved to me why optimum nutrition for athletic performance requires no more than a balanced diet composed of foods that are readily available at grocery stores and supermarkets. The only people who benefit from expensive supplements are those who sell them.

In 1971, I began eating a carbohydrate-rich diet with only moderate amounts of proteins and fats (60%–20%–20%). By 1972, I was in the best shape of my life. In April of 1972, I won the Collegiate Mr. America bodybuilding contest.

A Text Worth Having

Dr. Eleanor Whitney was a faculty member at Florida State University in the 1970s, and I enrolled in one of her advanced nutrition classes. Dr. Whitney had an inspiring interest in publishing, and she excelled at putting together educational materials based on nutrition science. Her college-level nutrition textbooks are by far the best on the market, and millions of copies have been sold.

My personal favorite is the 16th edition of *Nutrition Concepts and Controversies.* It contains 700 pages and several hundred charts, graphs, and pictures. It's the best scientific source on food and nutrition, and it's written in an entertaining style.

Discovering the Facts

When champion athletes attribute their outstanding speed, strength, or endurance to a food supplement, it's perfectly natural for other athletes or those participating in serious fitness programs to pay attention. If a magic food, pill, or dietary regimen might change you quickly into a world champion, why not give it a try?

It may be natural, but it's still a mistake. I've interviewed athletes at three Olympic Games trained many world-class amateurs and professionals, but I've yet to meet a single such person who understands what happens to his favorite foodstuff after it enters the body. Such athletes obtain their results despite their nutritional beliefs and not because of them.

Intermittent Fasting

Intermittent fasting is popular today among some dieters and fitness-minded people. The idea involves consuming no food energy during some portion of a 24-hour day—usually 12, 14, or 16 hours.

Besides fat reduction, research shows that intermittent fasting daily for several months may reduce inflammation, reduce the chances of stroke, and improve conditions such as arthritis, asthma, diabetes, and multiple sclerosis. Interestingly, intermittent fasting can extend lifespan in rats.

Some of my trainees have been successful with a 12-hour fasting goal. The 12:12 plan is a workable option for beginners. They have a first meal at 7 a.m. and the last meal of the day at 7 p.m. In between are a small meal and a snack. Thus, there are 12 hours of food during the day and 12 hours of no food at night.

Calories still count, and they should total 1200 to 1600 per day. Overall, I like the 300–400 calorie breakfast, lunch, and dinner, plus a small snack. Staying well hydrated is important.

Going for the more aggressive 16:8 objective is tougher for most dieters. The 16:8 plan limits eating to an 8-hour window. Some guidelines say you can eat and drink whatever you want during that window with *no calorie restrictions*.

It's much smarter, in my opinion, to eat moderately during your meals. Consume a reasonable number of calories, and don't overeat.

Compared to any form of intermittent fasting, I prefer my tried-and-proved **Still Living Longer Stronger Eating Plan**, as described in chapter 22.

Food Supplements

A food supplement is a product in pill, powder, or liquid form consumed in addition to or in place of food.

It is illegal to market any product with therapeutic claims until satisfactory evidence of its safety and effectiveness has been presented to the Food and Drug Administration (FDA). Many nutritional products, however, are marketed for the prevention or treatment of a health problem. The therapeutic claim does not appear on the product label; instead, it is communicated to retailers and customers through books, pamphlets, or word of mouth. Promoters of these products call them supplements, hoping they will be considered foods rather than drugs and therefore be exempt from the laws regulating the sale of drugs.

Promoters of nutrition fallacies and scams are skilled at using myths to arouse fears and false hopes. Here are some of them.

- Myth 1: It is difficult to get the nourishment you need from ordinary foods.
- Myth 2: Vitamin and mineral deficiencies are common.
- Myth 3: Virtually all diseases are caused by inadequate eating.
- Myth 4: Most diseases can be prevented or treated by nutritional means.

None of these concepts is true. It has been well established that eating according to the recommended guidelines is more than adequate for the vast majority of adults.

Vitamin and Mineral Pills

People in the United States spend approximately $30 billion a year for vitamin and mineral supplements. Most people who use them believe they are getting nutrition insurance, but many also think that vitamins can provide extra energy, improve general health, and prevent disease. Those who take individual vitamins usually believe that these products have medicinal value in many areas.

Nutrition Insurance: Virtually all nutrition authorities agree that healthy individuals can get all the nutrients they need by eating a wide variety of foods. Most Americans believe this too, but at the same time many worry that their eating habits place them at risk for deficiency. This fear of not getting enough is promoted vigorously by food faddists and supplement companies. Too many people fail to understand that the RDAs are set high enough to encompass the needs of individuals with the highest requirements.

Perspectives on Food Processing: The supplement industry frequently promotes the idea that the processing of food removes much of the nutrients. This may be true to some degree, but usually the changes are not drastic. In fact, many processed foods have nutrients added to them to replace what was destroyed. Furthermore, processing can make foods safer, cheaper, and often tastier.

Stress Vitamins: Some manufacturers have advertised that extra vitamins are needed to protect against physical or mental stress. Typically, stress vitamins contain ten times the RDA for vitamin C and several of the B vitamins. Although vitamin needs may rise slightly in certain conditions, they seldom rise above the RDA. Even if they do, they can still be met by ordinary foods.

Natural Versus Synthetic Vitamins: Many companies claim that natural vitamins are superior to synthetic versions, and they charge more for what's natural. Scientists know that vitamins contain specific molecules and that your body makes no distinction between molecules made in nature and those made in laboratories.

Protein Supplements

For years, the biggest misconception among athletes was the belief that strength training and muscle-building exercise require massive protein intake. I wish I had understood the facts about protein and muscle-building before I spent thousands of dollars on various food products.

There is little muscle-building, performance, or health benefit from high-protein supplements. You can meet your protein needs by eating several small servings each day of meat and dairy products. The RDA for protein—0.36 grams per pound of body weight—is an excellent guide for adult men to follow. Thus, if you weigh 180 pounds, your protein need is 180 × 0.36, or 64.8 grams per day.

Appropriate Use of Food Supplements

In general, food supplements are useful only for people who are unable or unwilling to consume an adequate diet. For example, physicians often recommend various food supplements for:

- Very young children until they are eating solid food.
- Older children with poor eating habits.
- Children who do not drink fluoridated water.
- Pregnant teenagers, who are likely to need supplementary iron and folic acid.
- Pregnant women with a history of iron deficiency.
- Children eating vegetarian diets that do not supply enough vitamin B12.
- Individuals adhering to prolonged low-calorie diets.
- Individuals recovering from surgery or serious illnesses who have disrupted eating habits.
- Post-menopausal women who are prone to osteoporosis.
- Elderly individuals who lose interest in food and eating.

As you can see from the above listing, few of these descriptions apply to reasonably healthy women and men.

My Personal Supplements

At 80 years of age, my maximum heart rate has decreased significantly, and my metabolism has slowed. I no longer eat the number of dietary calories that I could in my 50s. My body systems are not as efficient as they once were. Thus, I do take a few food supplements.

One person has been primarily responsible for the supplements I consume.

From 1985 to 1988, my right-hand man at Nautilus was Tim Patterson. Tim was in his mid-30s and was the most committed worker I've ever been around. No job was too small nor too big for him. "Tim: organize this; plan that; get an appointment with this person; write a page on the latest machine." Tim did it all—thoroughly, honestly, and quickly.

When Nautilus was sold and disassembled for the third time in 1989, Tim relocated to Colorado Springs, Colorado, and I moved to Gainesville, Florida. But we continued to talk and do small projects together.

Tim did some promotional work for Dr. Michael Leahy, a chiropractor with a concept called Active-Release Techniques. I set up an office at the Gainesville Health & Fitness Center, where I started training and doing studies with interested club members.

Several years passed, and we were both busy. Tim visited the publisher of a magazine called *Muscle Media 2000* and had some inspiring conversations with the owner, Bill Phillips, and the chief editor, TC Luoma. Phillips and Luoma were also manufacturing and promoting food supplements under the name of EAS.

Problems occurred at *Muscle Media 2000*, and Phillips and Luoma parted ways. Patterson hired Luoma, and they started a publishing company called T-Nation and eventually a food supplement business called BioTest.

With the emergence of the Internet in the late 1990s and early 2000s, Tim and I were both active and thriving. Tim lent his steady hand to help me prepare and market two books: *Living Longer Stronger* (1995) and *A Flat Stomach ASAP* (1998). Then he helped me organize a website.

Tim has also applied his thorough, honest approach to his food supplement business.

As a result, for more than twenty years, I've taken the following products, which are manufactured by Tim Patterson under the BioTest label:

- **Metabolic Drive:** A protein powder made from micellar casein and whey isolate.
- **Flameout:** A fish-oil softgel that contains Omega-3 fatty acids.
- **ZMA:** A zinc/magnesium capsule.
- **Surge:** A carbohydrate-rich workout fuel (recently developed) with electrolytes in powder form.

The supplements listed above have found a welcome place in my day-to-day living.

III

REMOVING EXCESS BODY FAT

Still Living Longer 13 Stronger

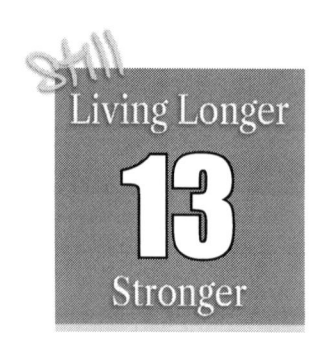

Patterns of Fat Distribution

Men and women store fat differently. Men tend to deposit fat in the front of the body, particularly the abdominal region. Women tend to deposit fat in the back of the body, especially the buttocks and upper thighs.

Another genetic difference is that men tend to store more of their fat on the trunk rather than on the arms and legs, as women do. Much of the adipose tissue that a man accumulates on his front will be around the navel and over the sides of the waist. *Pot belly* and *love handles* are the familiar terms used to describe these conditions.

A Personal Experience

As almost everyone who has gone on a typical reducing program knows, you seem to lose weight from everywhere else first before it finally starts coming off your midsection. I know from my own attempts to lose fat that it comes off my love handles last.

My normal body weight is 178 pounds, which includes the familiar love handles that I don't like. If I carefully work on a few things for several months and get my weight down to 170 pounds, my waist will be two inches smaller, but those love handles are still there.

Only when I get down to 168 pounds do those stubborn fatty deposits disappear. But I don't like how my face looks at 168—so I try to be satisfied at somewhere between 170 and 178 pounds.

It's a cruel trick of nature that we tend to lose fat last from the very places we'd like to lose fat the most. There's a reason for this, however, that is related to the fat cells themselves.

Alpha and Beta Receptors

For a fat cell to be stimulated, it must have a receptor for nerve action.

Fat cells have two types of receptors, called alpha and beta. The alpha receptors increase fat storage, while the beta receptors stimulate the breakdown of stored fat.

Most men have fat cells in their abdominal areas that are rich in alpha receptors. In other parts of their bodies, the fat cells are rich in beta receptors. This helps explain why belly fat is difficult to remove. Most women have more beta receptors around their buttocks and upper thighs.

With the SLLS plan, I'm going to share many techniques for men and women that I've utilized over the years that will surprise you. Within your genetic potential, you'll be able to note some amazing changes in your waist, hips, thighs, and elsewhere.

Energy and Calories

Energy is the internal power you must have for everything you do:

breathing, sleeping, digesting, and exercising.

In your high-school physics class, you probably learned that energy cannot be created or destroyed. It can only change its form and the place where it is available.

The sun is the ultimate source of energy. Plants can grow by combining the energy from the sun with the elements from the air, soil, and water. Animals usually get their energy from plants. Humans get energy from plants and animals.

From a nutritional viewpoint, food and energy are measured in calories. One calorie (*kilocalorie* is the scientific term) is the amount of heat energy required to raise the temperature of one kilogram (a liter) of water by one degree centigrade. The calorie is the unit we use to express the energy value of foods, or the energy required by the body to perform a given task.

The energy values of foods are established by measuring the amount of heat given off when a specific amount of the food is burned inside specially designed equipment. After years of experimentation, scientists found that the figures below are suitable for estimating the amount of energy supplied by various mixed diets.

- 1 gram of carbohydrate = 4 calories
- 1 gram of fat = 9 calories
- 1 gram of protein = 4 calories

The calorie expenditures for various types of activity have been calculated and written up in many diet and exercise books. It is well known that activity burns calories, and that if you are on a diet with a calorie limit that doesn't meet your body's energy demands, your body will find the calories it needs from your fat stores.

Losing fat, however, is more than a matter of simple addition and subtraction. It is true that any diet that contains fewer calories than you expend will cause you to lose weight. But unless that diet contains the correct balance of carbohydrates, fats, and proteins, much of the weight you lose will not be from your fat stores. Instead it will come from the water stored in your lean body mass (your organs, blood, muscles, and bones). This is not where you want to lose weight.

Nutritionists have determined—and my research over the years has confirmed—that the ideal fat-loss eating plan should be balanced as follows: 50 percent carbohydrates, 25 percent fats, and 25 percent proteins.

14

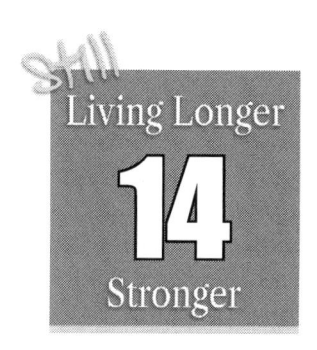

Still Living Longer Stronger

Losing Fat Through Your Skin

What happens to fat when you lose it? How does it get out of your body?

I often pose these questions to groups who are interested in fat loss. Judging from the responses I get, most people are baffled but intrigued by the science behind the correct answers.

When you understand the facts that follow, you can use them to make all your fat-loss actions more productive.

Little-Understood Ways We Lose Fat

Fat is energy, and energy is best expressed in calories. One pound of body fat contains 3,500 calories. No matter which energy system your body is using, it burns calories. Therefore, caloric intake counts significantly in losing fat.

Your body gets rid of fat or calories in three ways: through your skin, through your lungs, and through elimination of fluids as urine. Although you lose a small amount of heat through your feces, it is not thought to be significant unless you are suffering from diarrhea.

Most of the calories are eliminated through your skin. Your skin is our body's largest organ, and as much as 85 percent of your daily energy emerges through it as heat. You lose heat through your skin by radiation, conduction, convection, and evaporation.

Radiation

Heat radiates from the surface of your body. Whenever you are near something that is cooler than you are, heat leaves your body and is absorbed by that object. Or if the object is warmer, your body would absorb some of the object's radiant heat. Approximately 50 percent of the calories emitted through your skin each day are radiant heat.

A tall, lean person has a larger body surface area than another person who is the same weight but stockier and shorter. Because the tall person constantly loses more calories by radiation, he or she can consume more calories than the shorter person. Radiation is why shorter people tend to get heavier and taller people tend to remain lean.

Almost all your skin's surface emits calories through radiation. The exceptions are places where exposure is limited because one skin surface touches another, such as under your arms. But nature has compensated by increasing the number of sweat glands in those areas.

Conduction

Conduction of heat means the transfer of calories through direct contact. For example, when you get into a cold swimming pool, heat from your body immediately goes into the water. Water is a much better conductor than air, so you can lose more calories in cold water than in cold air. Conversely, if you are in a hot tub full of water with a temperature higher than your skin, calories will be conducted to your skin's surface.

Various substances have different capabilities to conduct heat. Air, being a poor conductor, can be used as an insulator. Much of the insulation in new homes today works by trapping pockets of air between walls. Clothing is generally a poor conductor; thus, it usually insulates and keeps us warm. But we all have experienced the difference between wearing cotton and wool.

One tip concerning conduction that I learned years ago, from talking with Olympic wrestlers, is that shivering burns three times as many calories as sweating. Before their final weigh-ins, these wrestlers were often frantic to lose that last half-pound of fat and qualify for a lighter weight classification. Shivering, they found, was the best way to accomplish this goal.

I've always encouraged my fat-loss groups to adapt their bodies to being uncomfortably cool as they progress. This can be accomplished in several ways, even during sleep.

Convection

Your skin disposes of another 15 percent of heat loss by convection. This means that air is circulating around your skin to move away the heat that has been formed by conduction. In other words, air movement helps with the elimination of heat. That's why the wind makes you feel cooler when you bicycle or walk, and it's why a fan overhead in a workout room cools you off as you exercise below it. It's also why, on windy days in winter, the "wind chill" is lower than the actual outside temperature.

Evaporation

Your skin perspires constantly—every second, day and night. You are probably not aware of it unless sweat beads up visibly on your skin. The reason you are not aware of it is evaporation.

At ordinary room temperature, the moisture vaporized and lost from your skin, plus that from your lungs, accounts for approximately 25 percent of the calories lost by your body at rest. One-third of the heat lost by evaporation is removed through your lungs, and the other two-thirds is lost from invisible perspiration on your skin.

Humidity, as anyone who lives in the South can testify, has a major effect on how efficient your skin is at cooling you by evaporation. As the humidity increases, the perspiration on your skin can't evaporate as quickly. That's why sports or workouts combined with high heat and high humidity can be dangerous. When the humidity is high, your body must depend primarily on radiation and convection to eliminate calories.

Strength Training Connection

How efficient your skin is at eliminating calories depends on the blood flow through it. Your skin, as well as being your largest organ, is also very vascular. It is filled with arteries, capillaries, and veins. As you shrink your subcutaneous fat, the vessels in your skin will become more prominent.

The main purpose of this large vascular supply is to enable your skin to control the removal of calories and thereby govern your body temperature. Here is where proper strength training comes into the picture.

There is no better way to train your skin than to exercise the underlying muscles. With proper strength training, you can isolate and work any part of your body—from the little muscles of your feet and hands to the large muscles of your thighs and chest—which pumps blood to those specific areas. This surging blood brings nutrients and heat that helps your skin look better. The rising heat in the muscle must then be released through your skin. And your skin learns to adapt better by becoming a more efficient heat regulator.

Two Other Ways

Besides losing fat or heat energy through your skin, you also transfer it through your lungs and through your urine.

Approximately 10 percent of your daily calories and heat loss go through your lungs. Your lungs act as a bellows. Inhalation brings in oxygen-rich air, which is vital for energy metabolism. Exhalation carries out oxygen-poor air and the waste product carbon dioxide.

The remaining 5 percent of your heat calories are lost through urine. In chapter 15, I'm going to describe how drinking more water and increasing your urine production aids fat loss.

Transition to Environment

Let's recap briefly.

What happens to fat when you lose it? You can neither create nor destroy energy; you can only transfer it. Thus, fat is converted to energy and transferred out of your body, where it is used by other living organisms and by the environment.

How does this energy get out of your body? Secondarily, it leaves through your lungs and urine, but primarily it leaves through your skin.

Your skin deserves your respect!

Still Living Longer 15 Stronger

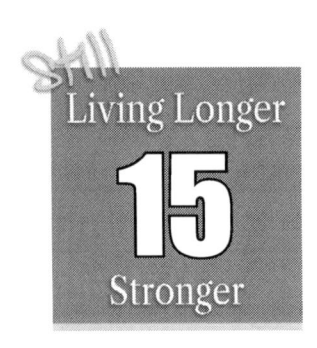

Watering Your Fat Away

Over the last forty years, I've written so much about the importance of consuming large amounts of water for fat loss that it's easy for me to take it for granted. So this is a good time to back up and review some of the key reasons why your body thrives on water and how that relates to fat loss.

First Things First

During my initial fat-loss work at Gainesville Health & Fitness back in 1985, I experimented by having some of my Nautilus Diet subjects consume ice-cold water to curb their hunger. It worked so well that I started recommending that their daily water—which now had been increased to 1 gallon a day—be consumed chilled. It wasn't long before hundreds of women and men, throughout GHF, were carrying insulated water bottles to their workouts and wherever else they traveled throughout the day.

When you drink water that's cooler than your body's core temperature (about 98.6 degrees Fahrenheit), your body must raise the temperature of that water to 98.6 degrees before it can eliminate the excess as warm urine. It just made sense to me that drinking ice water would burn more calories than room-temperature water (more on this later in the chapter). And, as weeks passed, I could see the overall results of the group that was consuming chilled water were better than the group that wasn't.

In 1988, I coined the word *superhydration* to mean the almost continuous sipping of 1 gallon, or more, of ice-cold water per day to boost the rate of fat loss.

In 2003, it was nice to see peer-reviewed research from Germany, by Dr. Michael Boschmann and colleagues, which reinforced my own protocols.

Your Water Is Showing

The adult human body is 50 to 65 percent water. But not all body components have the same water percentage. Your blood, for example, is 83 percent water, your brain is 75 percent, your muscle is 72 percent, your skin is 71 percent, your bone is 30 percent, and your fat is 15 percent.

As your body experiences dehydration, you feel it first in those systems that contain the most water. For example, you lose your mental alertness, and you suffer from overall muscular weakness. The last component that dehydration affects is your fat. That's why excessive sweating makes almost no dent in reducing your body-fat percentage.

Men have more water in their bodies than women, primarily because men have more muscle mass and less fat than women. A lean man with a body weight of 180 pounds may have 14 gallons of water in his system. A gallon of water (128 fluid ounces) weighs approximately 8 pounds, so simple multiplication (8 × 14) reveals that 112 pounds of this man's body is water.

You may not think of water as food, but it's the most critical nutrient in your daily life. You can live only a few days without it. Every process in your body requires water. For instance, it:

- Acts as a solvent for vitamins, minerals, amino acids, and glucose.
- Carries nutrients through the system.
- Makes food digestion possible.
- Lubricates the joints.
- Serves as a shock absorber inside the eyes and spinal cord.

- Maintains body temperature.
- Rids the body of waste products through the urine.
- Eliminates heat through the skin, lungs, and urine.
- Keeps the skin supple.
- Assists muscular contraction.

Water Your Fat Away

Increasing water intake facilitates the fat-loss process in several ways:

Kidney-liver function: Your kidneys require abundant water to function properly. If your kidneys do not get enough water, your liver takes over and assumes some of the functions of the kidneys. This diverts your liver from its primary duty: metabolizing stored fat into usable energy.

If your liver is preoccupied with performing the chores of your water-depleted kidneys, it doesn't efficiently convert the stored materials into usable chemicals. Thus, your fat loss stops, or at least plateaus. Superhydration accelerates the metabolism of fat.

Appetite control: Lots of water flowing over your tongue keeps your taste buds cleansed of flavors that might otherwise trigger a craving. Furthermore, water keeps your stomach feeling full between meals, which can help take the edge off your appetite.

Urine production: Here's a little-understood fact: Roughly 8 percent of your daily heat loss is through warm fluid being passed out through the normal urination process. Superhydration can double, triple, or even quadruple your urine production. As a result, you'll be able to eliminate more heat. Remember, inside your body, fat loss means heat loss. So, get used to going to the bathroom more frequently than normal. If your urine retains much of its yellow color, you're not drinking enough.

Cold-water connection: Have you ever wished for a food that supplies negative calories? Let's say such a food exists and it contains –100 calories per serving. Anytime you feel like a piece of chocolate cake or a donut, all you do to cancel it out is simply follow the sweet with two servings of the negative-calorie food. Presto—200 calories plus −200 calories yields 0 calories. While there is no such thing as a negative-calorie food, ice-cold water has a similar, but smaller, effect inside your body.

When you drink chilled water (about 40 degrees Fahrenheit), your system must heat the fluid to your core body temperature, about 98.6 degrees. This process requires almost 1 calorie per ounce of cold water. Thus, an 8-ounce glass of cold water burns approximately 8 calories—7.69, to be exact. Drink 16 glasses (128 ounces, or one gallon), and you've expended 123 calories of heat energy, which is significant. There's real calorie-burning power in cold water.

A professor of biology at the University of Florida added to my understanding of the cold-water connection when he pointed out that melting ice and a burning candle both require the transfer of heat. In both cases, matter is being transformed from one phase to another. The ice changes from solid to liquid, and the candle from solid to gas. Both transfers, or exchanges, involve heat.

Constipation help: When deprived of water, your system pulls fluid for its cells from the contents of your lower intestines and bowel, creating hard, dry stools. One of the big roles of water in the body is to flush out waste. This is a substantial task during fat metabolism because waste tends to accumulate quickly. Superhydration tends to make people more regular and consistent with their bowel movements, which is helpful to the overall fat-loss process.

Noradrenaline, the fat-burner hormone: One of the main problems when trying to lose weight, especially around your belly, is getting those fat cells to "let go" of the fat. We now know that the stimulant hormone called noradrenaline unlocks the fat that's trapped inside your cells. Instead of just burning sugar for energy (and leaving your belly fat untouched), noradrenaline tells your body to start using belly fat for energy. So how can you get more noradrenaline into your system? Cool your body down from the inside by drinking ice-cold water.

Cold-Water Guidelines

How do you drink a gallon of ice-cold water a day? "With great difficulty," you may reply. Although such a recommendation may sound difficult, in fact it presents only a few minor problems: how, when, and where. Each of these problems can be solved with some intelligent preparation and careful planning.

Note: Anyone who has a kidney disorder or takes diuretics should consult a physician before trying superhydration.

How: One secret is to not gulp or guzzle the water, but to sip it. Get yourself one of those 32-ounce plastic bottles, the kind that has a long straw in the top. I've found that most people can consume water more easily with a straw than trying to gulp it down the standard way with a glass. Also, while you're checking out various bottles, select one that is insulated. The insulation will keep your fluid colder for a longer time.

When: Another tip is to spread your water drinking throughout the day. That said, try to consume 50 percent before noon and the rest before 6 p.m. so you aren't having to get out of bed during the night to visit the bathroom.

Several of our dieters have commented that getting up in the middle of the night to urinate leaves them with a feeling of dehydration. If that's a feeling you have, it's fine to drink 4 to 8 ounces of water before you go back to bed.

Another tip, used by patients on an overnight fast before surgery, is to suck some crushed ice. Doing so provides a feeling of coolness and moisture without providing an excessive quantity of water.

Where: You sip water everywhere you go during the day because you know how to plan. Once again, you need a 32-ounce insulated plastic bottle. Okay. But what about ice, refilling the bottle, and all that hassle of keeping count of the ounces?

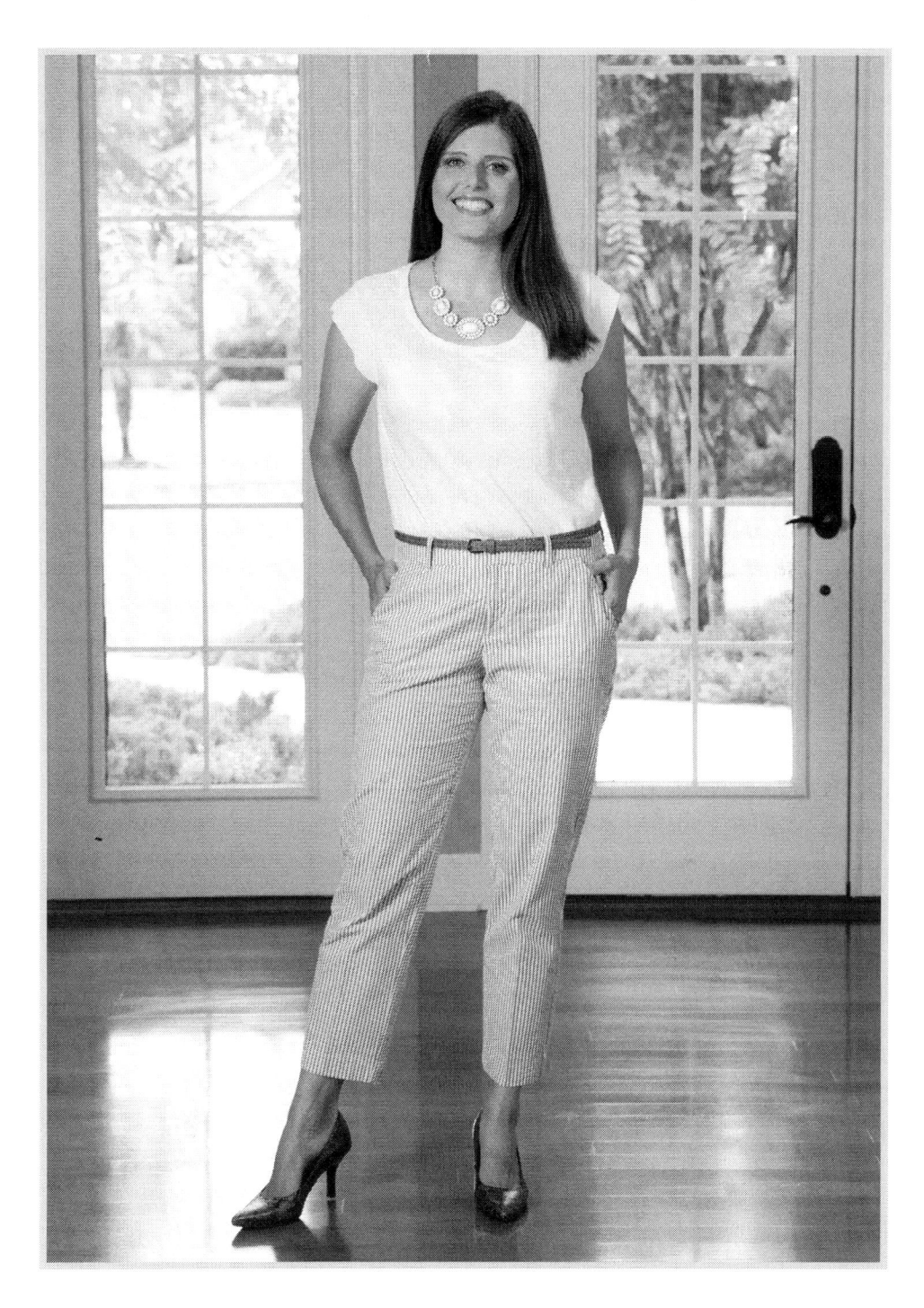

Melissa Jones, age 39, found it difficult to lose her pregnancy weight after having twins. The program helped solve her problem, as she lost 20 pounds of fat and built 7 pounds of muscle. "I give a lot of the credit to drinking the ice water," Melissa says. "It really keeps my appetite in check and benefits my muscles."

Some really motivated people invest in a 1-gallon insulated thermos jug. First thing in the morning, they fill the jug with ice and water. Then they draw off their initial 32 ounces of fluid into their insulated bottle and start sipping. As soon as the bottle is empty, it's refilled from the thermos jug. When they leave home each day, they carry both the thermos jug and the smaller bottle with them. That way they always have access to their chilled water. When they return home that evening, they thoroughly wash the jug and the bottle so they're ready for the next morning.

Some thermos jug designs are much easier to clean than others. Usually a larger cap, or a cap at both ends, makes cleaning easier. A little Clorox is a popular additive to ensure purity and prevent mildew from building up. As with shoes, having a second bottle and rotating their use allows more time for air-drying. One tip, if you fall behind, is to speed things up with a hair dryer.

A great way to keep count of the bottles and ounces is to place rubber bands around the middle of the bottle equal to the number of bottles of water you are supposed to drink. Each time you empty the bottle, take off a rubber band and put it into your pocket. Four 32-ounce bottles equal one gallon, so if a gallon per day is your goal, you'll need 4 rubber bands. Four beads on a knotted string would be another system, like a rosary.

Additives

There is a difference between plain water and other beverages that contain mostly water. Those mostly-water fluids—such as soft drinks, coffee, tea, beer, and fruit juices—contain sugar, flavors, caffeine, and alcohol. Sugar and alcohol add calories. Caffeine, found in coffee, tea, and many soft drinks—stimulates the adrenal glands and acts as a diuretic, which dehydrates the body. Keep all such beverages to a minimum.

The only recommended flavoring for water is a twist of lemon or lime. Even people who like lemon or lime eventually get to the point where they prefer their water plain with nothing added.

Tap Water Or Bottled Water

The decision to consume bottled water, or not, is usually one of preference. Some considerations:

In general, municipal water supplies in the United States are among the safest in the world. Chances are high that your community's tap water is fine for drinking. Furthermore, research shows that bottled water is not always higher quality water than tap water. So, if you have no problems with your city's water supply, then save some money and consume it. If you are concerned about chlorine, leave your jug of tap water open on the counter for several hours before adding the ice, and the chlorine will evaporate.

If you dislike the taste of your tap water, then drink your favorite bottled water. Just be sure to check the label carefully for unwanted additives. Also be aware that many of the bottled waters are simply city water in a plastic bottle.

A Few Words About Plastic

Plastic is often used for water bottles and jugs because it's lightweight (which makes shipping less costly) and it doesn't shatter if dropped. However, questions have been raised about the safety of certain kinds of plastic used in bottles and jugs, particularly BPA (bisphenol A) and especially during the summer heat of the Sunbelt states. If this concerns you, look for BPA-free jugs and bottles. There has also been a trend towards stainless steel bottles, which are both food-safe and reusable. Keeping plastic bottles out of landfills is a selling point for these. Just be sure to clean them thoroughly each night with dish detergent, hot water, and a bottle brush.

Water: Does One Size Fit All?

Frequently, trainees in my groups ask me about my blanket recommendation to drink 1 gallon of ice-cold water a day. They want to know why the recommendation is the same for a 300-pound man and a 150-pound woman.

In 1996, for several fat-loss groups, I tried the following formula: 1 ounce of water for every 2 pounds of body weight. If you were 300 pounds (man or woman), you would begin with 150 ounces a day. On the other hand, if you were a 150-pound individual, you would start with 75 ounces. Every two weeks, you would recalculate the ounces per day based on your new, lower body weight.

This recommendation worked fine when I was dealing with individuals or small groups of 5 people or less. But in large groups of 20 to 30 individuals, both men and women, there tended to be some confusion. And when I compared the overall fat-loss results of groups that used the formula versus those that used the blanket recommendation of 1 gallon per day, there were no differences. They all had approximately the same fat-loss results.

So, for the Living Longer Stronger program, I have opted for the simplest guideline for men and women, big or small, young or old: *Drink 1 gallon of ice-cold water a day.*

Too Much of a Good Thing

It's possible to drink too much water, but it's highly unlikely that you would ever do so. Drinking too much water leads to a condition known in the medical literature as hyponatremia. Hyponatremia most often occurs in athletes involved in triathlons and ultramarathons. Occasionally one of these athletes will consume many gallons of water during these unusually long competitions, and because of the continuous activity, they don't or can't stop to urinate. Thus they impede their normal fluid-mineral balance and become intoxicated with too much water. This condition, however, is rare.

Some of my research participants have consumed up to 1½ gallons of water in a day, and I've never observed anything close to water intoxication happening with any of them. Of course, they also have no trouble urinating frequently.

Note: Anyone who has a kidney disorder or takes diuretics should consult a physician before trying superhydration.

Still Living Longer 16 Stronger

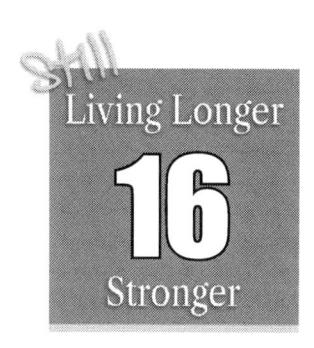

Eat a Meal, Walk a Mile

At one time, I was quick to pass off walking as an unserious method for losing fat. But because of a single study, I include it now as a valuable factor in my fat-loss formula.

A Salient Study

In the early 1990s, I discovered a study by Dr. J. Mark Davis and colleagues at the University of South Carolina's Department of Exercise Science. Dr. Davis measured and compared seven subjects for the calories burned for three hours after completing the following treatments: walking only, walking followed by a meal, and a meal followed by walking. He found that the meal-then-walking routine increased the calories burned among the participants by an average of 30 percent compared to the other treatments.

The university researchers concluded that going for a walk after you eat brings on "exercise-induced post-prandial thermogenesis." This simply means *the production of extra body heat created by exercising on a full stomach.*

Add Water to the Recipe

Other researchers have also studied the effect of walking after eating. They too found that taking a walk after a meal can speed up the production of heat, temporarily, by as much as 50 percent.

After reviewing that literature, I wondered: Had anyone studied the thermogenic effect of eating before a walk and then sipping ice-cold water *during* the walk? I could locate no references. But I discussed this concept with Dr. Michael Boschmann of the Medical Research Center at Humboldt University in Berlin, Germany, and he agreed with me that sipping ice-cold water during an after-meal walk would surely increase the heat produced.

Dr. Boschmann, if you recall from the last chapter, published the 2003 report "Water-Induced Thermogenesis" that reinforced my superhydration practices.

Eating-Walking-Sipping Routine

After working with more than 700 trainees at Gainesville Health & Fitness, here's the eating-walking-sipping routine that I have found most effective:

- Eat your evening meal. Plan to start your walk no more than 15 minutes after you finish eating.
- Put on lightweight, comfortable clothes and comfortable walking or running shoes (not street shoes).
- Fill an insulated bottle with 16 ounces of ice-cold water.
- Walk at a leisurely pace (about 3.0 miles per hour) for 30 minutes—not 29, nor 31, but exactly 30 minutes. Aim to cover 1½ miles in 30 minutes.
- Sip 16 ounces of cold water as you walk.
- Do the above each day for 42 consecutive days.

Calories Burned From Eating-Walking-Sipping Routine

Body Weight in Pounds	120	140	160	180	200	220	250	275	300
Calories burned by walking* at 3.0 mph for 30 minutes	96	111	127	142	159	176	200	219	246
+ 30% for walking after a meal	29	33	38	43	48	53	60	66	72
+ 15 calories for sipping 16 oz cold water during the walk	15	15	15	15	15	15	15	15	15
Total Calories Burned by the Eating-Walking-Sipping Routine	140	159	180	200	222	244	275	300	327

* Walking calculations are from the research of B.E. Ainesworth and colleagues, 2000.

Try my Eating-Walking-Sipping routine each day of the SLLS plan, and you'll be hooked on a leisurely walk after dinner as a healthy habit for life.

A Daily Walk for Your Head

As a subscriber to the *AARP Bulletin*, I recently read an article by Martha Murphy about walking and brain health, reported in the May 2023 issue.

Murphy's well-researched article says that walking may:

- Help you grow more brain cells.
- Boost your creativity.
- Enhance your mood.
- Reduce the risk of cognitive decline.
- Decrease brain-damaging stress.

Her push is to walk outdoors daily for 20 to 30 minutes.

That sounds familiar, doesn't it?

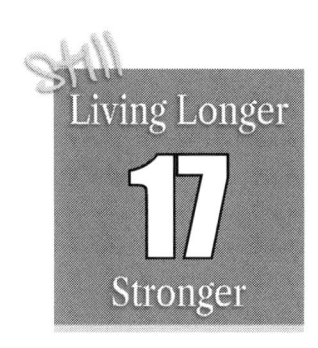

The Importance of Extra Sleep

Most people who are trying to fight fat need to grasp that at least 50 percent of daily fat loss occurs while they are sleeping. This is especially true for people on a 1,500-calorie-a-day eating plan combined with a rigorous exercise routine.

In addition to the diet and exercise plan, to make the entire SLLS program really work, I want you to focus on three important practices:

- Get at least 8½ hours of sleep a night . . . 10 hours is even better.
- Be less active during the day and night.
- Try to take a 30-minute afternoon nap.

What makes the above three practices so important is that they are based on science.

Dr. Artlet Nedeltcheva and his colleagues reported a study in 2010 in the *Annals of Internal Medicine.* The article was titled "Insufficient Sleep Undermines Dietary Efforts to Reduce Adiposity." Let's examine this research closely.

Sleep: A Powerful Fat-Loss Tool

The study compared two groups of overfat people who were each fed 1,450 calories per day for fourteen days. One group logged 8.5 hours of sleep per night, and the other clocked 5.5 hours per night (which, the authors noted, is the "norm" for most adults today).

After two weeks, the people who slept longer had lost significantly more fat than the group who slept less.

Most people who diet without utilizing strength training end up losing both fat and muscle. The same was true of the participants in the above-mentioned study on sleep and fat loss. But get this: The sleep-deprived group dropped 60 percent more muscle than the group who slept more. Those three hours of missing sleep caused a shift in metabolism that made the body want to preserve fat at the expense of muscle.

That was not all. When the researchers compared blood levels of appetite-regulating hormones in the two groups, they found that the subjects who slept less produced more of the appetite-stimulating hormone ghrelin. In other words, when they woke up, they were hungrier.

Many people assume that staying awake longer means their bodies burn more calories, but that is not the case. When sleep is inadequate, the metabolism slows down. In other words, when you sleep less, your body burns calories at a slower rate to preserve energy.

Here's another significant finding: On average, study participants burned *400 more calories by sleeping for three more hours.* That's an additional 2,800 calories per week, which is very significant.

With less sleep, the body seeks to meet the increased metabolic needs of longer waking hours by shifting into a lower gear that burns more muscle and less fat. Such is certainly not the type of fat-loss program that you want to be involved with.

In the final analysis, if you want to preserve muscle, burn fat, and wake up less hungry when dieting, sleep at least 8½ hours a night.

Lynn James

Age 61, Height 5' 8"

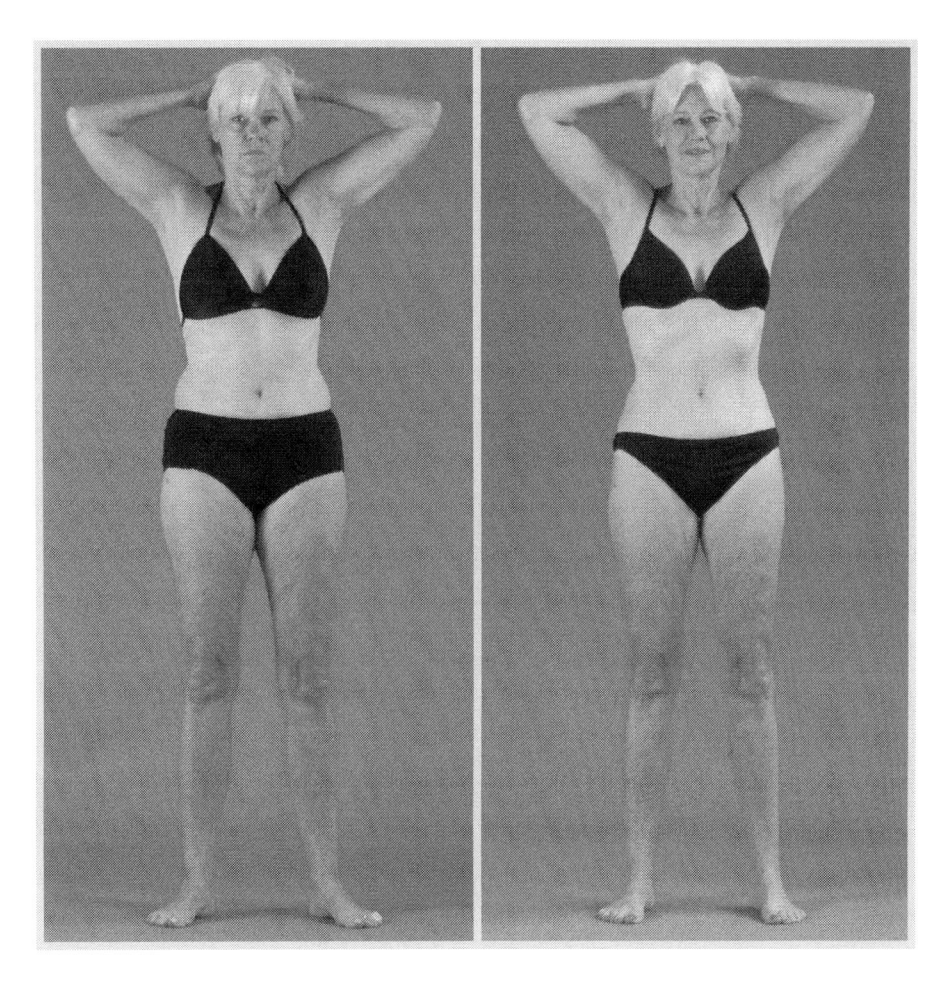

143 pounds   **131** pounds

After 6 weeks
15.25 pounds of fat loss, **5.125** inches off waist
5.375 inches off thighs, **3.25** pounds of muscle gain

"I only wanted to lose 5 pounds. Then, I started to sleep more and even take naps. Before long, this muffin top of mine is like GONE and I'm down 15 pounds. I'm so pleased."

Inactivity: A Powerful Muscle-Building Tool

Arthur Jones, the man who invented Nautilus strength training machines, explored for more than forty years the question: *If a muscle is stimulated to grow, when does it actually grow?* He could never boil it down to an exact time, but he did establish the following:

- Muscular growth, once it is stimulated, requires inactivity. Muscle will not grow if you are overly involved in various sports or fitness activities during non-training days. To make sure you get stronger, firmer muscles from exercise, you must rest more.
- More than 90 percent of muscular growth occurs during sleep—probably during a deep-sleep period of only 5 to 10 minutes.
- If in doubt about how much rest and sleep to get, err on the side of too much rather than too little.

During the research for my Body Fat Breakthrough program at Gainesville Health & Fitness, I observed some revealing behaviors among participants in the intense, negative-accentuated exercise program.

Negative-accentuated training increased participants' starting strength—their strength at the beginning of a workout—by perhaps 40 to 50 percent compared to normal training. It did this by triggering the production of at least six hormones: growth hormone, insulin-like growth factor, mechano-growth factor, interleukin-6, interleukin-15, and insulin.

The effects of these hormones on the human body were fatigue, the urge to rest, and deep sleep—and they all occurred *quickly*.

Such observations led me to the next research finding.

Naps Can Help Your Results

In addition to getting 8½ hours of sleep each night, I'm now asking you to take an afternoon nap. Yes, that's correct. Here's why.

Cheri Mah, MS, a researcher at the Stanford Sleep Disorders Clinic, asked members of Stanford's varsity basketball team in 2005 to try to sleep more. Every one of them did, and, in so doing, they improved their performance in sprinting, free-throw shooting, and three-point shooting.

Such findings eventually caught the attention of NBA players such as Steve Nash, Kobe Bryant, and Lebron James—all of whom slept more, liked it, and performed better. "Many athletes have optimized physical training and recovery," Mah wrote. "There really hasn't been the same emphasis on optimizing sleep and recovery."

The Stanford players and the initial NBA athletes were all encouraged to nap every day. Even a brief nap can help the body release crucial growth hormones that stimulate the healing of muscle and bone. To the athletes, the daily naps felt like a magic pill.

Enter Dr. Charles Czeisler, a professor at Harvard Medical School and today the go-to expert for professional sports teams from every major league. He noted that sleep deprivation could lead to high blood pressure, depression, and weight gain, as well as poor performances. What many athletes don't recognize is that it's the sleep after a game, or even an intense workout, that's most important.

Plus, Dr. Czeisler said that a 30-minute midafternoon nap could do wonders for recovery from sport activities. And that's precisely 30 minutes—no less and no more.

In my opinion, a midafternoon nap not only helps muscle recovery, it also contributes to fat loss. I've seen it with my own eyes many times.

For the Best Naps

If you've never napped, it may take a little effort. Here are four guidelines:

- *Time it right:* Try it between 2 and 4 p.m., the time your circadian cycle dips. Napping later in the day may make it more difficult to fall asleep at night.
- *Set an alarm:* Napping longer than 30 minutes may leave you groggy and disrupt nighttime sleep.

- *Nap in bed:* A cool, dark room will help you rest better.
- *Don't hit the snooze button:* When the alarm goes off, get right up. Walk around, splash water on your face, do a few jumping jacks—anything to wake you up and make you active again.

Rest More Now!

Follow the guidelines in this chapter, and not only will you enhance your resting and sleeping, but you'll also significantly improve your fat loss and muscle building.

18 Still Living Longer Stronger

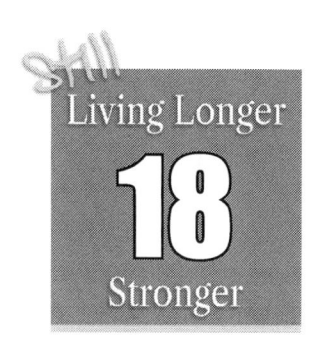

Hot News About Cold

Imagine a slumbering male black bear weighing 500 pounds, peacefully tucked away inside a cavern nestled among imposing mountains. Adorned with a dense fur coat and boasting a substantial layer of subcutaneous fat, this massive creature relies on those natural assets to regulate its body temperature during the arduous three-month winter.

As the winter gradually yields to spring and temperatures begin to climb, the bear stirs from its slumber, emerging from the cave with a gentle, unhurried gait.

Question: When it is not hibernating, how does this well-insulated bear manage to hunt, forage, and defend itself without succumbing to the perils of overheating?

For many years, this quandary perplexed Dr. H. Craig Heller and Dr. Dennis Grahn, biologists affiliated with Stanford University. Through persistent investigation, Heller and Grahn unraveled a fascinating truth. Bears have networks of veins near the surface of the skin on the hairless parts of their bodies. In thermal images of bears in the wild, most of the animal is practically invisible, but the pads of the feet and the tip of the nose appear ablaze because of how much heat they radiate.

Remarkably, most mammals have these networks of surface veins for radiating heat, and these veins are in different places depending on the animal: dogs have them in their tongues; elephants, in their ears; and rats, in their tails.

These surface vein networks allow more or less blood flow depending on the animal's need for cooling—from virtually none during frigid conditions to a substantial 60 percent of the heart's output during hot weather or vigorous activity.

A Cold Glove

Dr. Heller and Dr. Grahn found that in humans, these surface veins are primarily located in the face, the feet, and, most notably, the palms.

As a result of these findings, Heller and Grahn realized that the palms would be a good place to draw heat out of the body in medical situations where rapid cooling is needed.

Heller and Grahn devised a rigid plastic mitt or glove to place on one hand. Attached to the mitt was a hose that created a slight vacuum on the hand. The vacuum circulated cold water through the glove, and heat from the blood in the veins of the hand was rapidly carried away. The cooler blood then circulated through the rest of the body and cooled it by absorbing excess heat.

At first Heller and Grahn tested the glove during post-surgery situations to alter body temperature, which proved very effective in patients recovering from anesthesia.

Later, an athletic colleague used the glove to cool his hand between sets of all-out chin-ups on a horizontal bar. The glove seemed to erase muscle fatigue between sets.

The researchers then tried the cooling glove with other exercises, such as bench presses with a barbell, running, and cycling. In all individuals who used the cooling glove, muscles recovered their strength faster and soreness was eliminated.

But how does body temperature relate to muscle fatigue? Only recently was that answered.

Muscles and Heat Sensitivity

In 2009, researchers at Stanford determined that muscle pyruvate kinase—an enzyme muscles need to generate chemical energy—is extremely sensitive to temperature. At normal body temperature, the enzyme functions well. But as body temperature rises, the enzyme begins to deform into a non-functioning state. At a muscle temperature of 104 degrees Fahrenheit, enzyme activity shuts down completely.

As a muscle fiber works more intensely, it generates more internal heat. If too much heat were to build up, the fiber would self-destruct; in essence, it would cook itself and die. But muscle pyruvate kinase stops functioning before the critical temperature is reached. Without this enzyme, the muscle can no longer contract. But when you cool the muscle fibers, the enzyme returns to an active state, resetting the muscle's state of fatigue. So this enzyme called muscle pyruvate kinase is a crucial self-regulation system for our muscles.

You might be thinking: Instead of a high-tech glove, why not just stick your hand in a bucket of ice water?

That doesn't work well because it's so cold that it causes the blood vessels to shut down, meaning cooled blood is not transported to your core. Getting most of your body into a tub of cold water would circulate blood to your core, but often that's not practical.

A model of the Heller and Grahn glove is available commercially for $895. You should be able to locate information about this glove through Google on the Internet.

Some Cold Experiences

It was the first week of September 2012 when I first read the news from Stanford University about black bears, surface veins that radiate heat, and the cold glove. That wasn't the first time I'd heard about the benefits of getting cold, however.

At the 1972 Olympic Games in Munich, I heard that some Olympic wrestlers from countries in the Middle East were sleeping in cold environments, with no clothes nor covers, to lose a couple of pounds of fat before their official weigh-ins. These wrestlers said that being in an almost-shivering state consumed three times as many calories as sweating.

Ten years later, I read about a study in which subjects who got chin-deep in cold water lost fat faster. It worked because they were burning more calories than normal. Of course, these experiments were performed in a controlled environment with close medical supervision; this is not something people should try at home.

In 1985, based on those two bits of information, I recommended my fat-loss research subjects try keeping cool, as opposed to sweating, to burn more calories each day.

In 2008, Joe Cirulli, the owner of Gainesville Health & Fitness, told me about his first experience of submerging himself in his club's new cold plunge. Joe had heard good reports from a few fitness centers that put cold-plunge areas in their clubs. So, during his next club expansion, he put in a 100-square-foot cold plunge area in back near his swimming pool. It was specifically outfitted with the proper pumps and regulators to keep the water at 52 degrees Fahrenheit. Soon, many of his members loved taking a brief cold plunge after a hard workout. Most reported that the cold water seemed to eliminate many of their lower-body aches and pains. But Joe had not tried the cold water, and the area had been in operation for three months.

So, he developed a plan.

Cirulli and the Stadium Stairs

One of Joe's most grueling workouts involved going inside the University of Florida's football stadium and running up and down the stairs next to the tiered rows of seats. There were 80 rows of seats on the side that Joe ran, and he normally ran up and down five times. That always made his hips, thighs, and calves so sore that he had trouble sitting down for almost a week afterward.

His plan was to repeat the above routine with the addition of a cold plunge afterwards.

When the day came, he decided to really push himself by running up and down the steps seven times. By the time he made it back to his gym for the cold plunge, he could barely walk.

Upon entering the 52-degree water, he almost decided to bypass the ordeal. But a couple of friendly gym members joined him . . . and before he knew it, 10 minutes had gone by. Other members entered the cold plunge. Fifteen minutes had elapsed, then twenty. By that time, Joe's teeth were chattering, so he staggered out, took a hot shower, and drove home.

Once home, Joe said he had to put on a heavy coat, eat two bowls of hot soup, and drink a couple of cups of hot tea just to stop his shivering.

But guess what? When Joe got out of bed the next morning, he felt no soreness. There was no soreness the next day, nor the day after. *None*. Joe Cirulli hit a huge home run.

New Considerations

Joe's story sealed the deal for me. Beginning in February 2012, I decided to encourage all my fat-loss groups in Gainesville to take a cold plunge, for 5 to 10 minutes, after their negative-accentuated workouts. And, if a trainee could revisit the club and do the cold plunge one or two more times per week, that would be even better.

Approximately half of the first group of 55 subjects used the cold plunge at least once a week. The guy who did this most consistently was Herb Jones. And it showed.

Herb lost 35.96 pounds of fat and built 11.96 pounds of muscle over 6 weeks. He reduced his body fat to 8.5 percent, which was the lowest level of any participant.

The cold-plunge practice continued nicely from February through August. Then I read about the black bears and the Stanford research. Quickly, I had two ideas that could improve the results from the cold plunge at GHF.

First, all our trainees had been getting into the cold plunge at navel-deep level to start. After several minutes, they eased their torsos slightly deeper and endured for another 7 or 8 minutes. But the entire time was made more tolerable by keeping the hands and forearms completely above the water. Now, from reading about the Stanford research, I knew the effect on the overall recovery, as well as the calorie burn, would be more significant with the hands and forearms under the water.

Second, many of our trainees, before getting into the plunge, would put on a pair of these rubberized shoe socks to keep their feet a little warmer. I realized that these shoe socks were preventing the transfer of some heat from their feet to the cold water. So, no more rubberized shoe socks.

"Fat-Burning Fat"

"Fat-Burning Fat" was the subheading for a sidebar in Timothy Ferriss's 2010 book, *The 4-Hour Body.* The sidebar talked about brown fat, a special type of adipose tissue. I first read about the calorie-burning effects of brown fat more than thirty years ago. Brown fat is brownish in color and appears to be derived from the same stem cells as muscle tissue. This special fat helps get rid of excess calories as heat.

Black bears have a lot of brown fat over their necks and shoulders. Interestingly, humans store brown fat in the same places, though in much smaller amounts. In both humans and black bears, cold temperatures cause brown fat to burn regular subcutaneous fat at a higher rate than normal.

That's why, for accelerated fat loss, Ferriss recommended placing a U-shaped ice pack around the back of the neck and upper trapezius for approximately 30 minutes in the evening, three times per week. Several of my participants have tried this technique, and they seem pleased with the overall results. If you don't have access to a cold plunge, a U-shaped ice pack around the neck would be an alternative.

How About a Cold Shower?

Another suggestion from the Ferriss book involves the best way to take a cold shower—another substitute for a cold plunge.

- Use hot water for 1 to 2 minutes over the entire body.
- Step out of the hot water and apply shampoo to your hair. Lather up your head.
- Switch the water to pure cold and rinse your head and face alone.
- Turn around and back up into the cold water. Focus the spray on your lower neck and upper back.
- Maintain this position for 1 to 3 minutes. As you acclimatize, soap the rest of your body.
- Turn around and rinse.
- Exit the shower and towel yourself dry.

General Guidelines

Are there any additional scientific explanations for why the cold plunge seems to help muscle recovery?

To review, we have already considered the findings from Heller and Grahn concerning surface veins as well as the connection between muscle enzymes (pyruvate kinase) and internal temperature.

In general terms, cold minimizes micro-trauma in the muscle fibers. Subsequently, as the chilled tissue warms, the increased blood flow speeds circulation—which, in turn, makes the recovery process more efficient. Reducing the inflammatory process also seems to reduce the residual soreness traditionally associated with intense exercise, especially negative versions.

The advantage of submerging most of your body in cold water is that the entire surface area of the body, including over the major muscles, is subjected to cooling, rather than a small area covered by a localized ice pack.

Points to Practice

Personally, I've used the cold plunge multiple times, always with good results. Here are some additional guides to practice if you take the plunge:

- Be conservative with the water temperature. Most rehabilitation specialists recommend a water temperature of 54 to 60 degrees Fahrenheit. Gainesville Health & Fitness keeps their cold plunge at 52 to 54 degrees.
- Don't assume that colder is better. Spending time in water lower than 52 degrees can be dangerous. On the other hand, 60- to 75-degree water can still be beneficial.
- Keep your feet bare in the cold plunge. Do not wear rubberized shoe socks.
- Place your hands and forearms under the water.
- Stay in the cold plunge for 5 minutes initially. Gradually work up to 7 to 8 minutes. Do not exceed 10 minutes.
- Ease out of the cold plunge and wait 5 minutes before you shower.

IV

REBUILDING AND REDUCING PROGRAMS

19 Still Living Longer Stronger

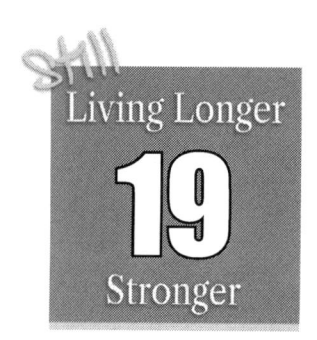

A 28-Pound Fat/Muscle Makeover

How would you like to lose 18 pounds of fat and build 10 pounds of muscle at the same time?

That's exactly what Richard West did in three months at 66 years of age. Richard is married and the father of two adult children.

At 5' 10" tall and a starting body weight of 195.5 pounds, Richard had been suffering from low-back pain, sore knees, and arthritis in his hands. These maladies limited his ability to golf, an activity he loved. As a leading divorce attorney in Orlando, Richard spent a lot of time sitting, which did not help his situation.

Richard responded agreeably to the SLLS eating plan, but it was the strength training workouts where he really excelled. He learned how to execute each exercise in focused form, and his 10-10-10 style was precise.

His body began changing for the better. Over three months in 2019, Richard added 3.5 inches on his chest and 2.25 inches on his upper arms, and he subtracted 3.5 inches from his waist. Plus, he dropped 18 pounds of fat. He's now playing golf without a hitch, and his low back and knees are secure, strong, and performing well.

Richard's *after* photo on the next page is one of the best in the book. You can really see his 28-pound fat/muscle makeover.

He is now a rest-of-his-life believer in strength training and the 10-10-10 method.

Richard West

Age 66, Height 5' 10"

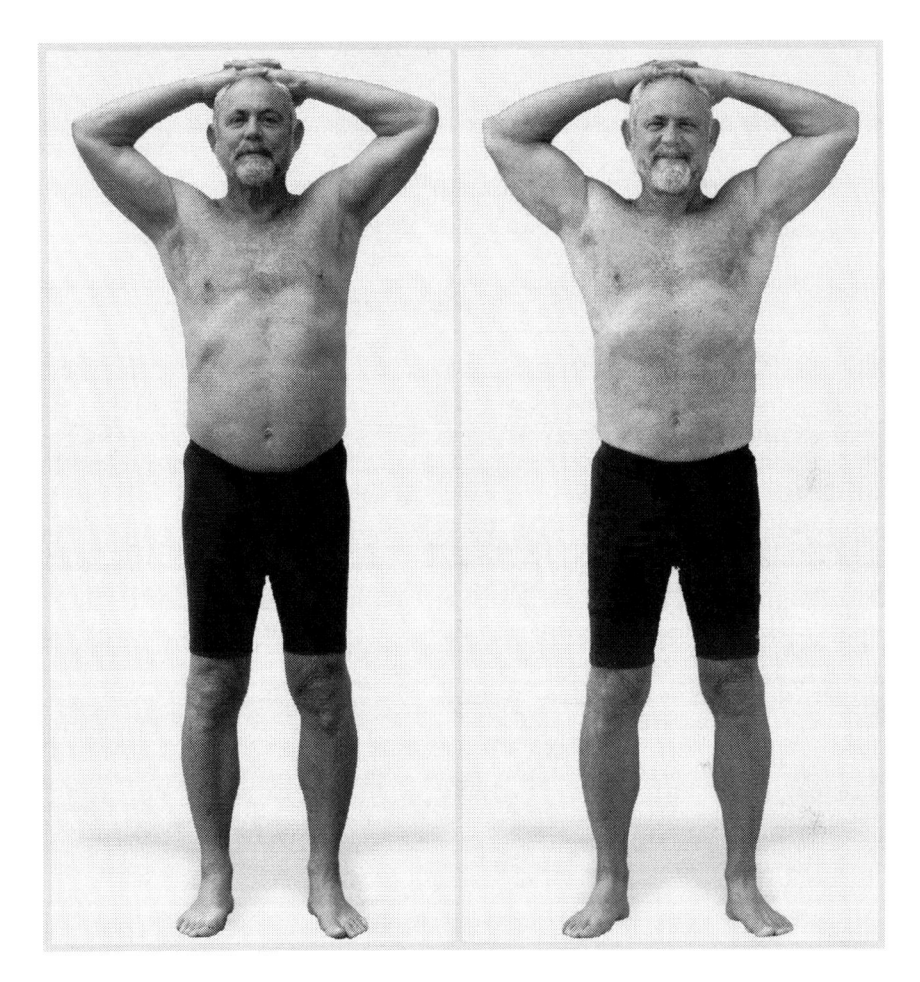

195.5 pounds   **187.5** pounds

After 12 weeks
18.36 pounds of fat loss, **3.5** inches off waist
3.5 inches added to chest, **2.25** inches added to upper arms
10.36 pounds of muscle gain

"I have several doctors I've seen for many years. And I have close friends who I visit on a regular basis. All of them are amazed at my makeover—and none of them can believe my weekly workouts require only 20 minutes. That weekly workout, however, has transformed my body and enhanced my life."

Still Living Longer 20 Stronger

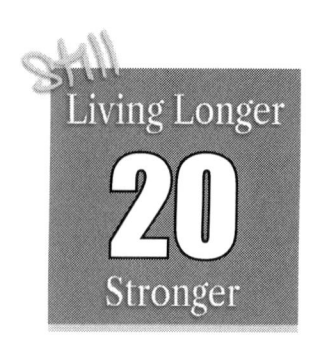

Before Getting Started

You probably already know that you have some pounds and inches to lose and some muscle to gain. But you probably don't know how to put a number—a realistic number—on what you want to occur throughout your body.

We discussed earlier that there's a difference between losing weight and losing fat. And most people need to lose fat specifically, not just weight. Determining just how much requires that you put a number on your own fatness. In this chapter I'll show you how to estimate your fatness with a simple test.

In six weeks, will your new body weight accurately reflect the new you? Only in a very general way. It is best to take full-body photographs of yourself, *before* and *after*, and compare them with your weight and circumference measurements. I'll show you what I mean by this later.

Do not skip the steps in this chapter! Take measurements and photographs before you begin the Still Living Longer Stronger plan. You'll be glad you did when the pounds and inches start melting away.

Follow the measuring instructions carefully so that your comparisons will be valid. Be precise and be consistent.

One note: It's difficult to take your own measurements accurately. You'll get truer numbers if you have a dependable partner or friend to help you.

Check With Your Physician

Should you call your doctor and schedule a routine physical examination? Actually, because of the prevalence and hazards of obesity in this country, most Americans should get their doctor's permission to *not* exercise and to *not* diet. There is, certainly, more risk involved in pursuing a sedentary, high-calorie lifestyle. Nevertheless, I recommend that you check with your physician before embarking on the program in this book. Take the book along with you for easy reference.

Some people should follow a certain program only with their physician's specific guidance. Consult your health-care professional beforehand and play it safe.

Record Your Height and Weight

Remove clothing and shoes and record your height to the nearest quarter inch and your weight to the nearest quarter pound. Be sure and use the same scale when weighing yourself at the end of the plan. For the most accurate results, weigh yourself nude in the morning.

Take Circumference Measurements

Before-and-after circumference measurements are meaningful because they let you know what is happening in specific areas of your body. Measure as follows, using a plastic tape measure:

Measurement	Where to measure	Tips
Upper arms	Midway between shoulder and elbow	Arms hanging and relaxed
Chest	Nipple level	Keep the tape level all the way around
Upper abdomen	Two inches above navel	Belly relaxed

Measurement	Where to measure	Tips
Mid-abdomen	Navel level	Belly relaxed
Lower abdomen	Two inches below navel	Belly relaxed
Hips	At maximum protrusion of buttocks	Feet together
Thighs	High, just below the buttocks crease	Legs apart, weight distributed equally on both feet

Body-Part Measurements

	Before	After	Difference
Height (nearest quarter inch)			
Body weight (nearest quarter pound)			
Right upper arm (hanging, in middle)			
Left upper arm (hanging, in middle)			
Chest (at nipple level)			
Two inches above navel			
At navel level			

	Before	After	Difference
Two inches below navel			
Hips (at largest protrusion)			
Right thigh (just below buttocks crease)			
Left thigh (just below buttocks crease)			

Do the Pinch Test

You can get a fair estimate of your percentage of body fat by doing the pinch test.

The pinch test for both men and women requires taking two measurements: on the back of the upper arm, and beside the navel. Here's the procedure to follow:

1. Locate the first skin fold site on the back of the right upper arm (triceps area) midway between the shoulder and elbow.
2. Let the arm hang loosely by the side. Grasp a vertical fold of skin between the thumb and first finger. Pull the skin and fat away from the arm. Make sure the fold includes just skin and fat and no muscle.
3. Measure with a ruler the thickness of the skin to the nearest quarter inch. Be sure to measure the distance between the thumb and the finger. Sometimes the outer portion of the fold is thicker than the flesh grasped between the fingers. To avoid this, make sure the fold is level with the side of the thumb. Do not press the ruler against the skin. This will flatten it and make it appear thicker than it really is.

4. Take two separate measurements of the triceps skin fold thickness, releasing the skin between each measure, and record the average of the two.
5. Locate the second skin fold site, which is immediately adjacent to the right side of the navel.
6. Grasp a vertical fold of skin between the thumb and first finger and follow the same technique as previously described.
7. Take two separate measurements of the abdominal skin fold thickness and record the average of the two.
8. Add the average triceps skin fold to the average abdominal skin fold. This is your combined total.

Estimate Percentage of Body Fat

Estimate your percentage of body fat from the chart below and record it on page _____.

Skin Fold Thickness	Fat Percentage	
Triceps + abdominal	**Men**	**Women**
¾ inch	5–9	8–13
1 inch	9–13	13–18
1¼ inches	13–18	18–23
1½ inches	18–22	23–28
1¾ inches	22–27	28–33
2¼ inches	27–32	33–38
2¾ inches	32–37	38–43

Your body fat percentage multiplied by your body weight equals the fat component of your body in pounds:

_____ × _____ = _____
Fat percentage   Body weight   Pounds of fat
from chart above   (before)   (before)

At the end of six weeks, weigh yourself again and repeat the pinch test. Refer again to the chart above to find your new estimated fat percentage. Then multiply that percentage by your new body weight:

_____ × _____ = _____
Fat percentage   Body weight   Pounds of fat
from chart above   (after)   (after)

Now, subtract as shown to see how much fat you've lost:

_____ − _____ = _____
Pounds of fat   Pounds of fat   Pounds of fat
(after)   (before)   lost

For example, if a woman weighed 168 pounds with 28 percent body fat at the start of the program, that's 47.04 pounds of fat. If she completed the program at 150 pounds at 18 percent body fat, that's 27 pounds of fat. The difference between 47.04 and 27 is 20.04 pounds; she has lost 20.04 pounds of fat.

Calculate the amount of muscle gained by subtracting your total weight loss from the fat loss:

_____ − _____ = _____
Pounds of fat lost   Weight loss   Pounds of
                                                  muscle gained

Continuing the example above, where fat loss equaled 20.04 pounds and weight loss was 18 pounds, 2.04 pounds of muscle were gained.

Fat composes more than 25 percent of the body weight of most Americans. An ideal amount of body fat for most men is 12 percent.

The average woman's ideal status is 18 percent. Lean, athletic men and women may desire to lower their ideal figures by another 5 or 6 percentage points.

Pinch-Test Measurements

	Before	After	Difference
Right Triceps			
Right Abdominal			
Total			
Body Fat Percentage			
Fat Pounds			

Take Full-Body Photographs

There is no better way to evaluate your current condition than to have full-body photographs taken of yourself in a small, revealing bathing suit. Digital cameras are easy to use. Here are the best procedures to follow:

- Wear a solid color bathing suit or bikini.
- Stand against an uncluttered, light-colored background.
- Have the person with the camera move away from you until he/she can see your entire body in the viewfinder. It's best to be 15 to 20 feet from the subject and zoom in with the camera lens. The photo should be in portrait orientation (vertical) rather than landscape (horizontal). It's also best for the photographer to be seated with the camera approximately 3 feet off the floor.
  Consider marking your position and that of the photographer with masking tape so you can be the same distance apart when you take your *after* photos.

- Have your assistant take three photos of you:
  1. **Front:** Stand facing the camera with your feet 8 inches apart. Interlace your fingers and place them on top of your head, so the contours of your torso will be plainly visible. Do not try to suck in your stomach.
  2. **Back:** Now turn so your back is toward the camera. Maintain the same pose: hands on your head, feet 8 inches apart, belly relaxed.
  3. **Side:** This time, you'll stand with your feet together (to get a better shot). Turn to one side (it doesn't matter which; just remember to pose on the same side when you take your *after* photos). Keep your hands on your head—remember, feet together this time—and keep that belly relaxed.
- Download the digital *before* photos to your computer, if necessary. Crop the best ones tightly into 4-inch by 6-inch sizes.
- Retake the photos six weeks later, following the same directions, with the same bathing suit, camera, and lighting.
- Crop and make the prints the same size as the *before* ones. Your height in both sets of photos should be precisely the same so that more valid comparisons can be made.

Achievable Goals For Those Under 65

Taking your *before* measurements and full-body photographs will help you determine realistic goals for your SLLS plan. The success stories throughout this book will also help.

The following averages provide specific pounds and inches lost and pounds of muscle gained. They were compiled from before-and-after measurements of 142 people (54 men and 88 women) who went through one or more phases of the course at Gainesville Health & Fitness.

Free Gift

Download the Still Living Longer Stronger 6 Week Program to enter all of your measurements.

livingstrongermethod.com/gift

Average Changes After 6 Weeks	
For men:	**For women:**
27.5 pounds of fat lost	15.5 pounds of fat lost
8 pounds of muscle added	4.6 pounds of muscle added
5.1 inches off waist	4 inches off waist

The people in Gainesville were handpicked by me, and they were extremely motivated, or they didn't last long under my disciplined coaching. Some, in fact, decided to leave after two weeks. Also, the average age was 46.

More Realistic Goals For Those 65 to 80

I believe more realistic goals for people 65 through 80 years of age are 70 percent of the numbers above. In other words:

Realistic Goals For Age 65 to 80	
For men:	**For women:**
About 19 pounds of fat loss	About 10.5 pounds of fat loss
About 5 pounds of muscle gain	About 3 pounds of muscle gain
3.5 inches off waist	2.8 inches off waist

These numbers provide realistic goals for second-middle-aged men and women motivated to follow the SLLS plan for six weeks. Some individuals will achieve lower results, while some can achieve greater results—as much as 75 percent above these numbers.

Some like Lynn James in chapter 17, wanted to lose only 5 pounds of fat. But 5 pounds led to 10, and 10 led to 15. "My body surprised me," Lynn remembers, "and my smile just keeps getting bigger and bigger."

So, be realistic, but don't be afraid to push your goals a little . . . or a lot.

Still Living Longer 21 Stronger

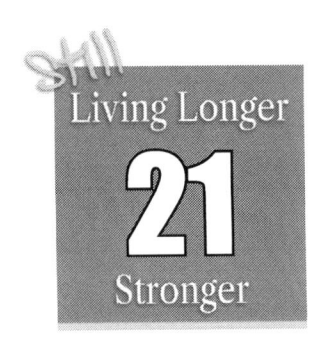

Overview of the SLLS Eating Program

One of my favorite sayings seems appropriate here: "If you fail to prepare, prepare to fail."

Here are a few more important steps to take in preparation for the SLLS eating program.

Purchase Measuring Spoons, Cups, and a Small Scale

Most people underestimate the size of one ounce of cheese, two ounces of chicken breast, or four ounces of orange juice. Such practices lead to inaccurate calorie counting and ineffective fat loss. It's important to use measuring spoons, cups, and food scales, and use them correctly.

All these items can be purchased inexpensively at your local supermarket, or department store. With the food scale, however, you'd be wise to spend more money and buy a battery-operated digital scale instead of the less expensive spring-loaded type.

Take a Vitamin/Mineral Tablet Each Day

During the program, I recommend that you take one multivitamin with minerals tablet each morning with breakfast. Make sure no nutrient listed on the label exceeds 100 percent of the Recommended Dietary Allowance. High-potency supplements are not necessary.

Examine the Menus, Recipes, and Shopping Lists

Glance through the SLLS menus, recipes, and shopping lists in chapter 22 for a view of what you'll be eating during the next six weeks. Your results will be more effective if you plan ahead.

Follow the Carbohydrate-Rich, Descending-Calorie Eating Plan

There are a few specific groups of people who should not try a reduced-calorie eating plan: children and teenagers; pregnant women; women who are breastfeeding; men and women with certain types of heart, liver, or kidney disease; diabetics; and those suffering from some types of arthritis and cancer. If in doubt, show this book to your doctor before proceeding.

Remember, carbohydrates are your body's primary source of energy as well as an important source of many vitamins and minerals. On the SLLS plan, approximately 50 percent of your daily calories are from carbohydrate-rich foods. The remaining 50 percent of the calories are equally divided between proteins and fats. This 50:25:25 ratio of carbohydrates, proteins, and fats is ideal for maximum fat loss and muscle gain. With slight modifications, this ratio can be continued for a lifetime of healthy eating.

Many overfat men and women make the mistake of immediately reducing their dietary calories from a typical 3,000 to 1,200 or fewer a day. Such a drastic cut in calories can cause at least three problems:

- First, after several days you may get an uncontrollable appetite, which causes you to break the diet.
- Second, a drastic reduction in calories may cause your body to preserve its fat stores.
- Third, your body starts conserving energy and burns fewer and fewer calories. As a result, you'll have to reduce your calories even more to keep losing.

Such extremely low-calorie diets are doomed to self-destruct.

I've found through my research that you can prevent these problems by reducing your calories in a gradual manner. That's exactly what the SLLS program does.

During Weeks 1 and 2, men start with 1,600 calories per day and women begin with 1,400 calories per day. For Weeks 3 and 4, the calories drop to 1,500 per day for men and 1,300 per day for women. For Weeks 5 and 6, there's another reduction of 100 calories: 1,400 per day for men and 1,200 per day for women.

At 1,600 calories a day for a man and 1,400 calories a day for a woman, you won't develop a ravenous appetite, nor will your body be stressed into a state of lowered metabolism. Quite the opposite will happen. Your body will become more efficient at burning fat.

Eat Smaller Meals More Frequently

You'll consume six small meals each day, with approximately 2½ hours between each meal. The only difference between the eating plans for men and women is that men add 100 calories to each Lunch and 100 calories to each Dinner selection.

The menus and recipes in the next chapter have all been simplified. The recipes are easy to cook and shop for. All you need to do is follow the easy-to-understand directions.

Drink 128 Ounces of Cold Water Each Day

Do not underestimate the importance of what I call superhydration, or drinking 1 gallon of ice-cold water each day. Invariably the individuals who lose the most fat in six weeks are the most consistent with their water drinking.

A 32-ounce insulated plastic bottle with a straw makes the process easier to follow. Most people find they can consume more fluid with a straw than they can by drinking from a glass. A great way to keep up with your superhydration is to place one rubber band around the middle of the bottle for each bottle you intend to drink. Each time you finish 32 ounces, take off a rubber band.

Do 10-10-10 Training Twice a Week

With the SLLS program, you'll exercise in the 10-10-10 style twice a week. Every two weeks, the calorie allowance goes down and the number of exercises in each workout increases.

Use the Cold Plunge After Your Workout

If you have access to a cold plunge after your 10-10-10 training, by all means use it for 5 to 10 minutes. If not, consider trying the U-shaped ice pack around your neck that I described in chapter 18. A cold shower, which I discuss in the same chapter, might even be an alternative.

Walk After Your Evening Meal

You'll burn more calories if you take a leisurely walk after your evening meal each day. Remember, you should begin the walk within 15 minutes after the evening meal and walk for 30 minutes only.

Sleep an Extra Hour Each Night

Getting extra sleep will absolutely help your fat-loss and muscle-gain results. The recommended way to get extra sleep is to retire an hour earlier each night but arise at the usual time each morning.

Avoid Overstress

You want to stay clear of extreme behaviors. Send as many messages as you can to your body that everything is okay, standard, and tranquil. Do not get stressed out. Stay calm. Under such conditions, you will freely pull calories from your fat cells.

Be Patient . . . Look Forward to Your Great-Looking Body

You are now well prepared to begin the SLLS program.

The next six weeks will make a difference in your life. Be patient.

Don't be surprised if, six weeks from today, everybody around you is talking . . . talking about your great-looking body!

Overview of the SLLS Eating Program | 157

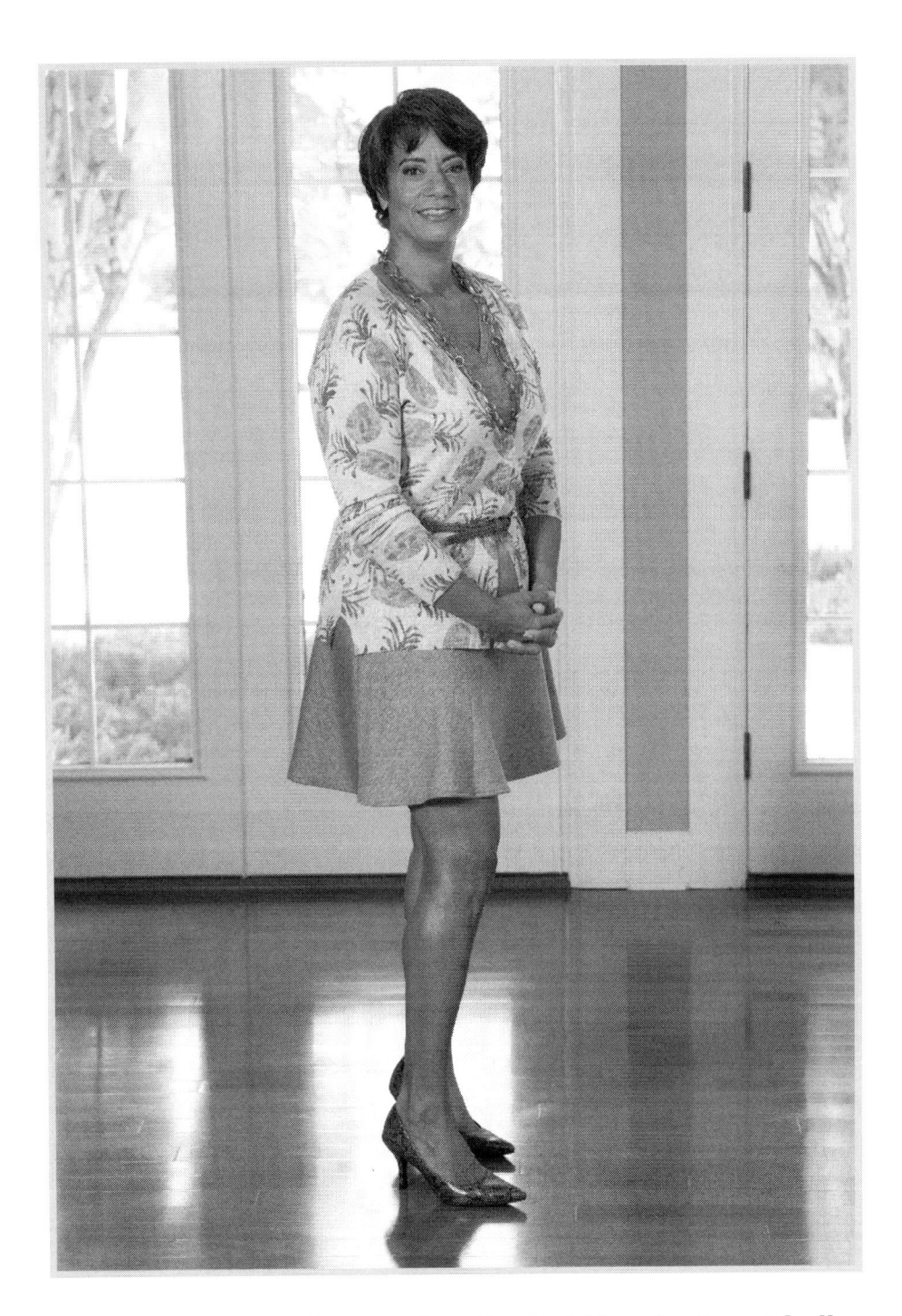

Nellie Otero, age 48, was skeptical at the start, not believing that Dr. Darden's program of working out less, sleeping more, and drinking lots of water would work. But that all changed. "I'm shocked at the results. Over 6 weeks, I lost 17 pounds of fat and gained 5 pounds of muscle. He made a believer out of me because I'm the proof."

22

Still Living Longer Stronger

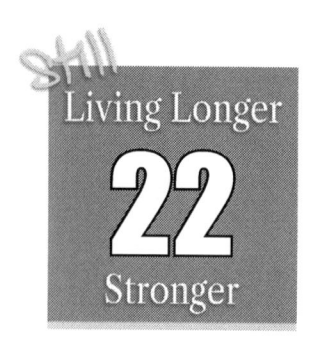

The Still Living Longer Stronger Eating Plan for Weeks 1–6

The menus in the eating plan are designed for maximum fat-loss effectiveness. For best results, follow them exactly.

Every attempt has been made to keep current the popular brand names and calorie counts, which are listed in the menus. But as you probably know, products are sometimes changed and discontinued. If a listed product is not available in your area for whatever reason, you'll have to substitute something similar.

Become a label reader at your supermarket. Don't be afraid to ask questions about food products. Supermarket managers are usually very helpful. If they don't have the answers to your questions, they will find someone who does.

Each day you will choose a limited selection of foods for breakfast and lunch. I've found that most adults can consume the same basic breakfast and lunch for months with little or no modification. Ample variety during your evening meal, however, will make daily eating interesting and enjoyable.

Additionally, the eating plan includes a midmorning, mid-afternoon, and late-night snack to keep your energy high and your hunger low.

Begin Week 1 on Monday and continue through Sunday. Week 2 is a repeat of Week 1. Calories for each food are noted in parentheses. A shopping list follows at the end of the chapter.

General Guidelines for the Menus

- Each daily menu consists of six small meals. A small meal contains from 100 to 400 calories. During Weeks 1 and 2, women consume 1,400 calories per day and men eat 1,600 calories a day. The listed foods are available in most supermarkets and are easy to prepare.
  Note: During Weeks 3 and 4, the calories drop to 1,300 per day for women and 1,500 per day for men. For Weeks 5 and 6, there's another reduction of 100 calories: 1,200 per day for women and 1,400 per day for men.
- The only difference between the eating plan for women and men is that men add 100 calories to each Lunch selection and 100 calories to each Dinner selection.
- *Noncaloric beverage* means any type of water—tap, bottled, carbonated, or flavored—with no calories. Soft drinks with zero calories count as noncaloric also. It's okay to have 1 or 2 cups per day of coffee or tea with caffeine—but no more than 2 cups.
- For the latest frozen microwaveable meals, and for possible Dinner substitutions, please refer to the following websites:
  - Michelinas.com
  - Healthychoice.com
  - Leancuisine.com
- For recommended meal-replacement shake mixes, see:
  - Metabolic Drive (MetabolicDrive.com)

Menus, Weeks 1 & 2

Women consume 1,400 calories a day; men consume 1,600 calories a day. Dinner is where the difference lies.

Breakfast = 300 calories

Choose one—bagel, cereal, or shake—and a noncaloric beverage.

  1 100% whole-wheat bagel, toasted, such as Thomas' (250)
  1 ounce light cream cheese (60)

1¼ cups Kashi GO Cereal (200)
½ cup fat-free milk (45) or
1 cup almond milk (40)

2 scoops of Metabolic Drive shake mix, Vanilla or Chocolate (220) or another meal replacement shake mix with a similar calorie count.
1 large banana (8¾" long) (100)
12 ounces cold water
Place in blender and mix until smooth.

Midmorning Snack = 100 calories

Choose one:

    1 cup light, fat-free flavored yogurt (100)
    14 whole unsalted almonds (100)
    1 apple (3" diameter) (100)
    2 cups light microwave popcorn (100)

Lunch = 300 calories

Choose one—sandwich or soup—and a noncaloric beverage.

    Ham or Turkey Sandwich (300)
        2 slices whole-wheat bread (140)
        1–2 tablespoons classic (yellow) mustard (0)
        3 ounces deli-type ham or turkey, sliced thin (90)
        1 ounce (1½ slices) fat-free cheese (50)
        2 slices tomato (10)
        2 lettuce leaves (10)

One 16.3-ounce can Campbell's Well Yes! Black Bean with Red Quinoa soup (280)

Men add 100 calories:
8 ounces original V-8 juice (45) and
7 whole unsalted almonds (50)

Midafternoon Snack = 200 calories

Choose two:

- 1 cup light, fat-free flavored yogurt (100)
- 1 Breakstone's Cottage Doubles, any flavor (100)
- 14 whole unsalted almonds (100)
- 1 apple (3" diameter) (100)
- 2 cups light microwave popcorn (100)

Dinner = 300 calories

Choose one frozen microwaveable meal and a noncaloric beverage.

- Butternut Squash Ravioli, Lean Cuisine Protein Kick (300)
- Chicken Teriyaki, Lean Cuisine Balance Bowls (310)
- Glazed Turkey Tenderloins, Lean Cuisine Protein Kick (300)
- Macaroni & Cheese, Michelina's (280)

Men add 100 calories:
1½ slices whole-wheat bread (105)

Evening Snack = 200 calories

Choose two:

- 1 cup light, fat-free, flavored yogurt (100)
- 1 Breakstone's Cottage Doubles, any flavor (110)
- 14 whole unsalted almonds (100)
- 1 apple (3" diameter) (100)
- 2 cups light microwave popcorn (100)

Substitutions for Weeks 3 & 4, Weeks 5 & 6

Women: Weeks 3 & 4 = 1,300 calories a day: Eliminate one Midafternoon Snack (–100 calories) from Weeks 1 & 2 Menus.

Weeks 5 & 6 = 1,200 calories a day: Eliminate one Evening Snack (–100 calories) from Weeks 3 & 4 Menus.

Men: Weeks 3 & 4 = 1,500 calories a day: Eliminate one Midafternoon Snack (–100 calories) from Weeks 1 & 2 Menus.

Weeks 5 & 6 = 1,400 calories a day: Eliminate one Evening Snack (–100 calories) from Weeks 3 & 4 Menus.

One of the Following May Be Substituted for a 300-Calorie Lunch During Weeks 3-6

Chef Salad
In a large bowl, mix the following:
2 cups lettuce, chopped (20)
2 ounces white-meat chicken or turkey (80)
2 ounces fat-free cheese (100)
4 slices tomato, chopped (28)
1 tablespoon fat-free dressing (8)

1 slice 100% whole-wheat bread, toasted (70)

Sandwich from Subway
6" Turkey Breast & Black Forest Ham on 9-Grain Wheat bread with plenty of raw vegetables; no oil-based dressings (300)

One of the Following May Be Substituted for a 100-Calorie Snack

Fruits
5 dried prunes (100)
1 ounce raisins (82)
½ cantaloupe (5" diameter) (94)

Energy Bars
Most of the popular energy bars—such as Powerbar, Kind, and Clif—may be used as snacks. Their calories, however, range from 210 to 240, so slightly less than ½ bar constitutes a 100-calorie snack.

One of the Following May Be Substituted for a 300-Calorie Dinner

Tuna Salad (220)
In a large bowl, mix the following:
1 5-ounce can chunk light tuna in water (100)
¼ cup (2 ounces) whole kernel corn, canned, no salt added (30)
2 tablespoons sweet pickle relish (40)
1 tablespoon Hellmann's Light Mayonnaise (50)
1 tablespoon Dijon mustard (0)

Mahi-Mahi and Broccoli (295)
4 ounces mahi-mahi fish, grilled (120)
1 cup broccoli florets, sautéed in 1 teaspoon olive oil (70)
1½ slices 100% whole-wheat bread (105)

Santa Fe–Style Rice & Beans, Lean Cuisine Protein Kick (310)
Creamy Rigatoni with Broccoli & Chicken, Michelina's (280)
Sweet & Sour Sauce with White Chicken & Rice, Michelina's (310)
Roasted Turkey Breast, Lean Cuisine Market Collection (290)

Shopping List for Weeks 1 & 2 Menus

The quantities for one week of the listed foods will depend on your specific selections. Review your choices and adjust the shopping list accordingly. Remember to check nutrition information on products you buy so that you can carefully follow the serving sizes in the menus. It may be helpful for you to photocopy this list each week before doing your shopping.

Staples

mustard
meal replacement shakes
fat-free milk or almond milk
whole, unsalted almonds
noncaloric beverages: water, diet soft drinks, tea, and coffee

Grains

Thomas' 100% whole-wheat bagels
Kashi GO Cereal
100% whole-wheat bread
light microwave popcorn

Fruits

apples (3" diameter)
bananas
dried apricots

Vegetables

lettuce
tomatoes
V-8 Juice (Original)

Dairy

light cream cheese
fat-free cheese
Light (low-fat), or fat-free flavored yogurt
Breakstone's Cottage Doubles

Meat and Entrees

white-meat turkey, thin sliced
ham, thin sliced
frozen microwaveable entrees
- Butternut Squash Ravioli, Lean Cuisine Protein Kick
- Chicken Teriyaki, Lean Cuisine Balance Bowls
- Glazed Turkey Tenderloins, Lean Cuisine Protein Kick
- Macaroni & Cheese, Michelina's
- Campbell's Well Yes! Black Bean with Red Quinoa Soup (16.3 ounce can)

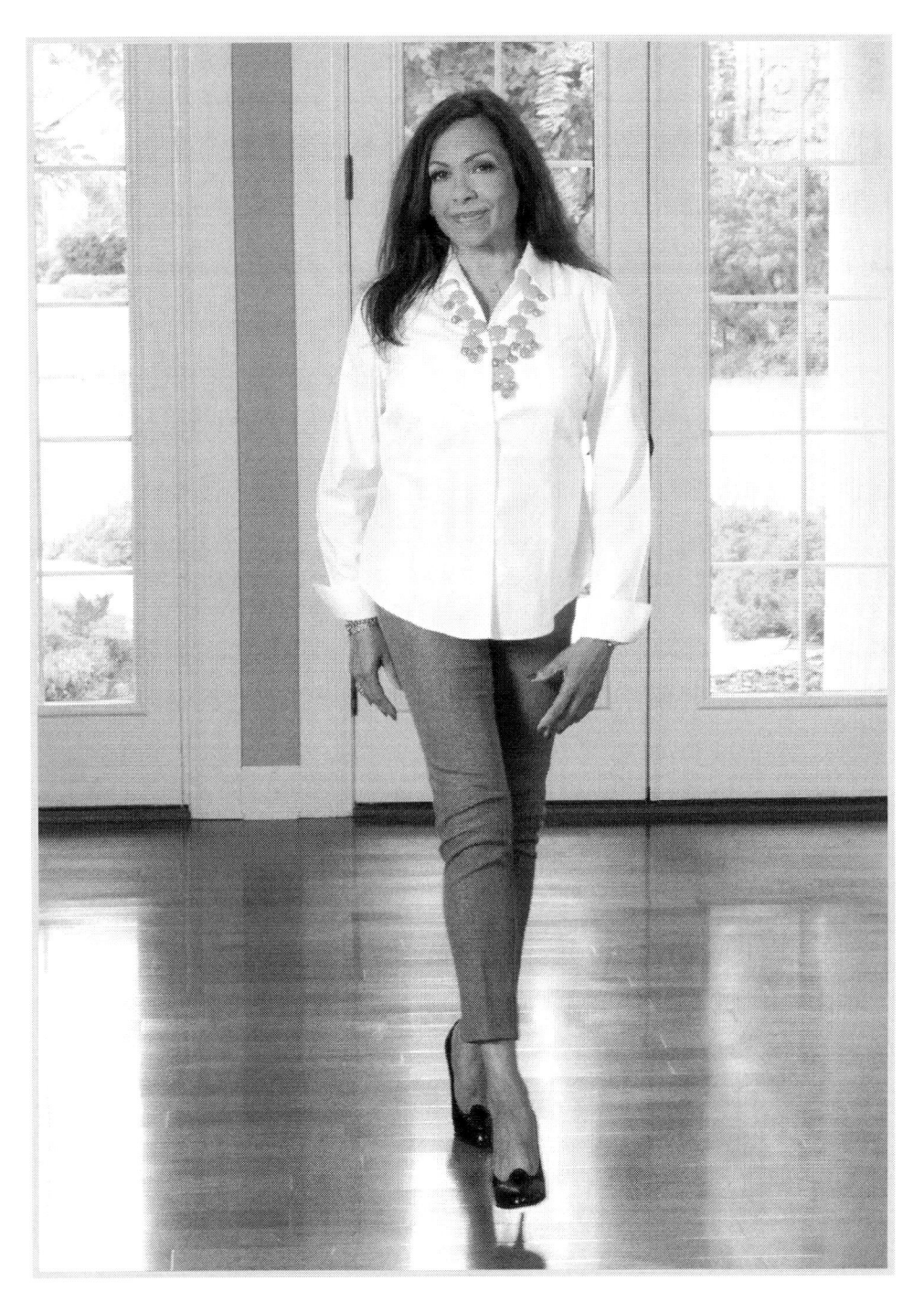

"I never dreamed," said Marlene Hill, age 59, "that I could lose 13 pounds of fat and 2.5 inches off my waist in 14 days."
You can read Marlene's story in chapter 28.

23

Still Living Longer Stronger

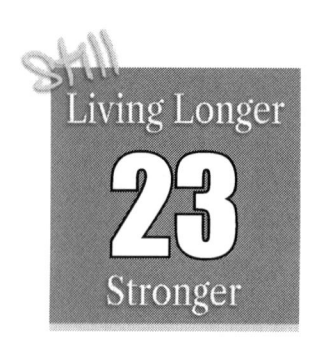

Living-Longer-Stronger Workouts For Weeks 1–6

Muscle-building exercise is an important component of the Living Longer Stronger Plan. From previous chapters you should be convinced that negative-accentuated training is the best type of muscle-building exercise for fat loss. Larger, stronger muscles aid fat loss by uniquely requiring more calories when you are at rest as well as at work.

Precision Guidelines

Read before you start: Spend several minutes looking over the exercises listed in the various routines in this chapter. Each exercise is detailed and illustrated in chapter 9 or 10, so you'll want to refer back to them frequently.

Choose between barbell-dumbbell movements and weight-machine exercises: If you train at home, you may want to use barbell-dumbbell movements. If you belong to a commercial fitness center, or gym, you'll probably have access to various weight machines. Most of the women and men involved in the SLLS research used weight machine exercises.

Select the appropriate resistance: Initially, it's important that you learn how to perform the exercises correctly. You'll learn better if the resistance is neither too heavy nor too light. Try to select a moderate resistance at first, something you can do easily for 10-10-10: 10 seconds on the negative, 10 normal reps, and 10 seconds on the final negative. After the first week, increase the resistance so that 10-10-10 becomes more challenging.

Control your movements: Rushing each exercise diminishes results and can cause injury. Keep a watch or big clock with a second hand in plain sight so you can move for the number of seconds indicated.

Count the seconds of each stroke: Record the actual number of seconds you make with each phase. When you can do 10-10-10, increase the resistance by 5 percent at the next workout.

Expect some soreness: Soreness in exercised body parts is an indication that you've stretched and contracted little-used muscles. Expect some soreness after each of your workouts, especially the ones that involve new exercises.

Keep your frequency: The idea is to do less as you get stronger. The frequency during Weeks 1–6 is twice a week, which means a training session on Monday and Thursday, or Tuesday and Friday.

Barbell-Dumbbell Routines

The following barbell-dumbbell routines are designed for use at home. They were also tested on small groups of exercisers at Gainesville Health & Fitness. They work well in both situations.

The routines are divided into three phases: Weeks 1 & 2, Weeks 3 & 4, and Weeks 5 & 6. The eight 10-10-10 exercises that use dumbbells are described in chapters 9 and 10.

Weeks 1 & 2

1. Squat With Dumbbells
2. One-Legged Calf Raise
3. Overhead Press With Barbell
4. Bent-Over Row With Barbell
5. Bench Press With Barbell
6. Biceps Curl With Dumbbells

Weeks 3 & 4

1. Squat With Dumbbells
2. One-Legged Calf Raise
3. Overhead Press With Barbell
4. Bent-Over Row With Barbell
5. Bench Press With Barbell
6. Biceps Curl With Dumbbells
7. Triceps Extension With One Dumbbell*

Weeks 5 & 6

1. Squat With Dumbbells
2. One-Legged Calf Raise
3. Overhead Press With Barbell
4. Bent-Over Row With Barbell
5. Bench Press With Barbell
6. Biceps Curl With Dumbbells
7. Triceps Extension With One Dumbbell
8. Shoulder Shrug With Barbell*

* New exercise

Weight-Machine Routines

For these routines, you'll need access to some basic exercise machines—such as Nautilus, Cybex, Hammer, or MedX—which are found in fitness centers throughout the United States and Canada. Where there is a choice of exercises, alternate between them, or use exclusively one or the other. Here are the recommended routines:

Weeks 1 & 2

1. Leg Curl
2. Leg Press
3. Chest Press
4. Lat Machine Pulldown
5. Triceps Extension With One Dumbbell
6. Abdominal Crunch

Note: The weight-machine exercises are described in chapters 9 and 10.

Weeks 3 & 4

1. Leg Curl
2. Leg Extension*
3. Leg Press
4. Chest Press
5. Lat Machine Pulldown
6. Triceps Extension With One Dumbbell
7. Abdominal Crunch

* New exercise

Note: The new exercise listed in Weeks 3 & 4 is described in chapter 9.

Weeks 5 & 6

1. Leg Curl
2. Leg Extension
3. Leg Press
4. Chest Press
5. Lat Machine Pulldown
6. Triceps Extension With One Dumbbell
7. Biceps Curl With Barbell*
8. Abdominal Crunch

* New exercise

Note: The new exercise listed in Weeks 5 & 6 is described in chapter 9.

Living Longer Still **24** Stronger

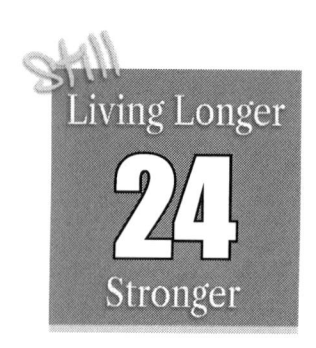

Troubleshooting Guide

During the first month of any new eating and exercising plan, certain situations may arise that cause hesitancy, doubt, and recrimination. For example, there was concern among the subjects about the prevalence of frozen microwaveable meals. Some asked why low-carbohydrate diets aren't an option. Common questions included how to deal with holiday parties and eating out at restaurants.

The following troubleshooting guide will help you prepare for these and other challenges to your progress.

Frozen Microwaveable Meals

Numerous magazine articles and books would have you believe that processed foods are bad for you. Processing, they claim, sacrifices many nutrients, and the added chemicals may be dangerous. Most foods, however, especially vegetables and fruits, are packed naturally with chemicals. "Chemical" can mean many things, not all of which are bad.

Recently, scientists at the University of Georgia and the University of California at Davis, in separate studies, found that frozen vegetables and fruits are just as nutritious as their fresh counterparts. In fact, the California research revealed that vitamin content was higher in some frozen foods, including broccoli, corn, green beans, and blueberries. The freezing process keeps the nutrients of harvested food intact, while fresh produce may sit in transport or supermarkets for days, losing nutrients along the way.

I have no financial arrangement of any kind with Lean Cuisine or its parent company, Nestle, who introduced Lean Cuisine and called it the healthier alternative. Some of their products are changing their name from *Lean* Cuisine to *Life* Cuisine. Since the late 1980s, I've used Lean Cuisine meals (as well as Healthy Choice, Michelina's, and Weight Watchers) as choices in my diet programs. I've consistently found Lean Cuisine to be tasty, varied, nutritious, economical, and adaptable to my daily macronutrient breakdown of 50 percent carbohydrates, 25 percent proteins, and 25 percent fats.

Today, Lean Cuisine has more than a hundred frozen selections, classified under breakfasts, lunches, and dinners, which you can review on their website, LeanCuisine.com. Most Lean Cuisine selections are between 250 and 400 calories, and you can absolutely trust their calorie counts. Also, they have broadened their scope to include meals that are vegetarian, gluten-free, and free of preservatives and artificial flavors. Most Lean Cuisine dinners contain less than 500 mg of sodium.

Low-Carbohydrate Diets

Some of the Gainesville participants were into low-carbohydrate eating before they were selected for my programs, so there was concern. Generally, there are two schools of thought on food and the process of weight loss:

- *Calories count:* The first school contends that the law of conservation of energy governs weight loss. The calorie is the unit of energy. According to this law, the energy, or calorie value, of the food eaten minus the energy expended must equal the sum of the heat given off and the physical work done by the body.
- *Carbohydrates count:* The second school argues that certain food combinations—namely, diets in which some carbohydrates are replaced with fats and proteins—have special qualities that cause weight to be lost more rapidly than would have been predicted by the law of conservation of energy. Calories aren't a critical factor in this position.

Important: Anyone who appreciates science and examines the evidence from both schools of thought soon realizes that human metabolism must obey the law of conservation of energy—as does everything else in nature. Isaac Newton initially recognized conservation of energy in 1687, and numerous other scientists, such as Max Rubner, Wilbur Atwater, Francis Benedict, and Albert Einstein, repeatedly confirmed the validity of the concept in the early twentieth century.

All dietary calories—whether in the form of carbohydrates, fats, or proteins—do indeed count.

The Real Facts About Low-Carbohydrate Dieting

Low-carbohydrate dieting has some problems associated with it:

- The initial weight loss from a low-carbohydrate diet is mostly water, not fat. Without carbohydrates, the body quickly depletes the sugars (glucose and glycogen) stored in the muscles and liver. Each ounce of sugar carries with it three ounces of water. It's not unusual for a dieter's body to burn 2 pounds of stored sugar in the first four to five days. Thus, 2 pounds of sugar + 6 pounds of water = a reduction of 8 pounds, 75 percent of which are water. Such excessive fluid elimination can lead to dehydration, which makes it harder to lose body fat.
- With low-carb diets, the lost water weight is quickly regained once eating returns to normal and the glucose/glycogen stores are replenished.
- Many low-carbohydrate diet plans say the dieter may "regularly" consume unlimited amounts—3,000, 4,000, even 5,000 calories a day—of non-carbohydrate foods. This might sound like a fun benefit, but it rarely happens. Most people's stomachs feel full long before they can actually consume that much bacon, steak, or what-have-you. And if satiety doesn't kick in, boredom generally will. Even your favorite fatty, protein-heavy foods become monotonous after a while.
- There is no hard scientific evidence to support the notion that the *source* of the calorie, rather than the calorie itself, is the key factor in becoming leaner. Gorging on dietary fat and protein will only cause the body to accumulate more stored fat.

- Lack of carbohydrates combined with an emphasis on fat and protein leads to an unhealthy condition called ketosis. Besides producing bad breath, ketosis causes the body to pull nutrients from its muscles, heart, and other internal organs.
- The high fat content of most low-carbohydrate diets is harmful to the cardiovascular system.
- A high-protein diet is especially risky for patients with diabetes because it can speed up the progression of kidney disease.
- A diet without significant amounts of carbohydrates is not conducive to an active lifestyle. And it deprives the brain of its primary source of fuel, thus contributing to a feeling of fatigue, "brain fog," and even depression.
- Absent some external health restrictions, most overweight people cannot endure strict low-carbohydrate dieting longer than two weeks. The initial weight loss from the elimination of water, however, gives them a false sense of success. Many believe that if they had continued longer, they would have reached their goal. Thus, the low-carb diet appears to have worked for a time when in fact it didn't, and these beliefs continue to be reinforced.

Carbohydrates and Maintenance

Concerning fat-loss maintenance, according to a study reported in a 1998 edition of the *Journal of the American Dietetic Association*, people who successfully lost an average of 30 pounds and kept them off for five years did so by eating more—not less—carbohydrates.

On the one hand, there are some carbohydrate-rich foods—such as candies and regular soft drinks—that should be limited on a fat-loss diet. On the other hand, as most registered dietitians proclaim, "Any carbohydrate-rich food has a place on a reducing diet, if it's consumed in moderation with a variety of other nutrients." Both sides have merit.

I believe that a variety of carbohydrate-rich foods is essential for successful fat loss as well as maintenance. And carbohydrates are a key energy provider for productive 10-10-10 training, which is the catalyst in the entire fat-loss process.

Combating Holiday Calories

It seems like almost every month of the year contains a major holiday. As a result, you'll regularly be eating and drinking at locations out of your direct control. Here are four defensive steps to take:

- **Plan ahead, eat ahead.** If the festivity includes dinner, find out what is on the menu. If there are not enough good choices, or if dinner is served well past your normal mealtime, eat at home. Budget 100 to 200 calories for some polite eating at the party.
- **Limit alcohol intake.** Alcohol is one of the most calorie-dense foods. Alcohol also tends to be accompanied by snacks galore. As one's judgment blurs, there's more to drink and more to eat. Social drinking can significantly increase the number calories you ingest in a day. Can you still enjoy your party if you halve your alcohol intake? Never drink alcohol when you're thirsty. Quench your thirst with water. If you are having mixed drinks, drink the mixer every other round.
- **Say "no" gracefully but firmly.** Here's a trick for avoiding a mega-calorie offering while still flattering your host: Say it looks delicious but you're too full to eat it right now, and request the recipe. You must be firm. This won't be easy; others may try to tempt you and may even resent you for having restraint. Tell them you must fit into a new pair of jeans, or something else similar.
- **Cut calories when not at social functions.** During the most tempting festive seasons, trim a moderate amount from your daily breakfast, lunch, and dinner to make room for the treats. But never go below 250 calories in a meal, and never skip meals.

Eating Out on the SLLS Plan

In today's health- and fitness-conscious society, virtually no restaurant is going to be surprised by, or unprepared to accommodate, special dietary requests. You just need to know how to explain what you want. Here are the best ways to order a suitable meal:

- **Request that a large pitcher of ice water be placed on your table.** Drink water freely before, during, and after the meal.
- **Leave the menu unopened.** The purpose of the menu is to entice you to spend big, and restaurants really know how to sell the sizzle.
- **Choose a simple green salad without such garnishes as croutons and bacon bits.** Lemon juice, vinegar, or a low-calorie preparation is preferable to any creamy or oily dressing.
- **Select one or two vegetables with nothing added.** A plain baked potato is nearly always available. Other good choices are broccoli, cauliflower, and carrots.
- **Ask the waiter what kind of fresh fish is available.** Order a white fish and have it baked, broiled, or steamed, with nothing on it. Although chicken is acceptable to order, it is usually prepared earlier in the day with marinades that add extra calories.
- **Be very specific with your order.** Double-check that your waiter understands exactly what you want. Don't be afraid to send something back to the kitchen if it's not what you requested.
- **For dessert, have coffee or tea,** or at most some fresh strawberries or raspberries.
- **Reinforce your preferences with the waiter and the manager as you leave.** Make them aware of your specific likes and dislikes about the food and the service.

Find a Partner for Problems

Most people find it helpful to have a buddy they can talk to about the SLLS program as they progress through it. Your buddy—whether it is a spouse, a friend, a coworker, or a neighbor—should be someone who is happy to talk about your goals, your meals, and your workouts. Plan to talk, text, or email five minutes each day.

Even better, although it's not always possible, is having a partner who can do the program with you. Share this book, trade small talk, contribute experiences, and enjoy triumphs. What's better than experiencing the satisfaction of achieving your goal? Helping someone else do the same.

Backslide Forward

You may have adhered to the SLLS diet strictly for weeks. Then you wrecked it one day when you walked by a donut shop. Fifteen minutes later, you'd wolfed down a half dozen!

Or you may have been progressing nicely with your negative-accentuated routine. An emergency, however, caused you to miss two workouts.

Now you feel guilty. You broke the diet. You sloughed off on your exercise. You feel like you might as well forget the entire program and go back to your old ways.

Don't let yourself fall into this senseless, destructive trap. Guilt saps your motivation and confidence.

Furthermore, such thinking indicates only a short-term goal. True power revolves around the realization that permanent fat loss is a long-term project that is bound to have ups and downs.

Expect to backslide occasionally. You're only human, right? There is no disgrace in backsliding. The disgrace lies in letting a lapse get you so discouraged that you quit trying. You must keep moving forward.

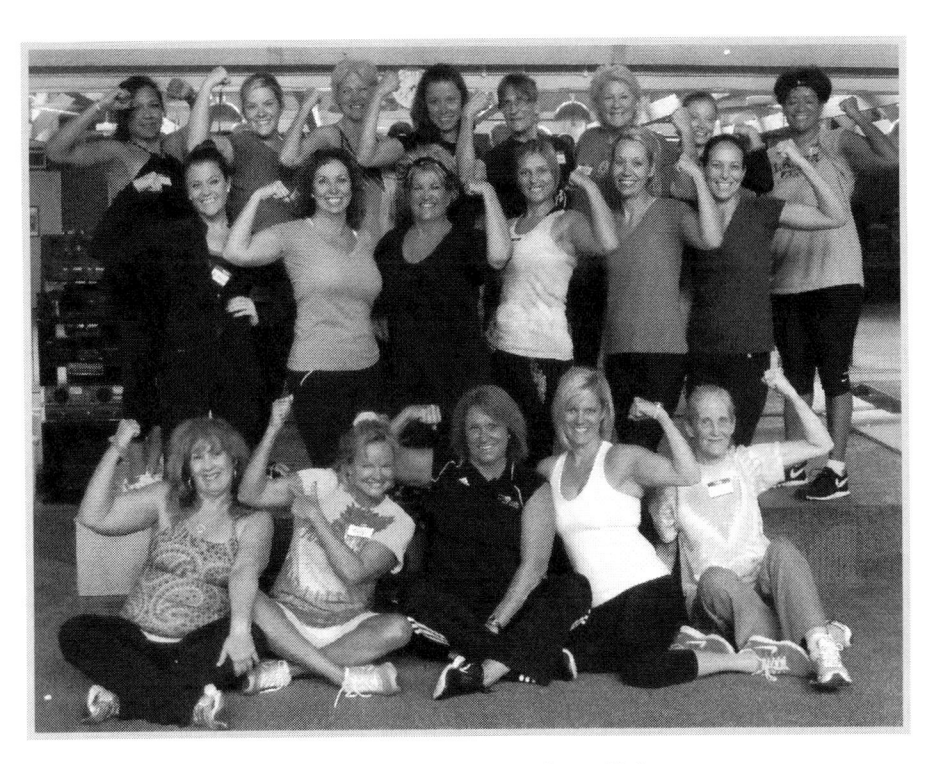

Here is a group of women who did my program at Gainesville Health & Fitness. You can see that they are proud of the muscles they built.

Body Weight Exercises

Several people have asked about doing strength training routines at home with only their body weight as resistance. Yes, this is possible, and a modified version of body weight exercises was applied at the Gainesville Health and Fitness with several groups. Below are the exercises that were performed:

Squat, for your hips and thighs: Stand with your feet shoulder-width apart. Hold your arms in from of your body at shoulder level. Lower your body smoothly by bending your knees and pushing your hips back. Try to get into a bottom position where the tops of your thighs are parallel to the floor. Push yourself slowly by straightening your knees back to starting position. Repeat for the required repetitions.

Wall Squat, for your hips and thighs: Lean back against a wall, with your feet 24 inches away from it and shoulder-width apart. Hold your arms in front at shoulder level. Slide your body down the wall until your thighs are parallel to the floor. Pause at the bottom and hold steady for a count of 30 seconds. That's your initial goal. Then, you can progress to 45 and then 60 seconds.

Hip Raise, for your hips and lower back: Lie face up on the floor with your knees bent and your feet flat on the floor. Place your arms out to your sides at 45-degree angles. Raise your hips so your body forms a straight line from your shoulders to your knees. Push against the floor with your heels and squeeze your glutes. Lower your body back to the floor. Repeat for the required repetitions.

Calf Raise, for your gastrocnemius and soleus muscles: Lean forward against a smooth wall. Your toes should be 2 to 3 feet from the wall. Rise on your toes as high as you can. Pause. Lower your heels slowly down to the floor. Repeat for the required repetitions.

Pushup, for your chest, shoulders, and triceps: Get face down on the floor. Place your hands under your shoulders. Set your feet close together. Straighten your arms and push up to the top position. Your body should form a straight line from your ankles to your head. Lower your body until your chest nearly touches the floor. Push yourself back to the top position. Do not let your hips sag during lowering or pushing.

Crossed-Arm Crunch, for abdominals: Sit on the floor with your knees bent and your feet flat on the floor. Cross your arms in front of your chest. Raise your head and shoulders and crunch your rib cage toward your pelvis. Pause. Slowly return to the starting position.

Plank, for your abdominals: Assume a pushup position, but bend your elbows and rest your weight on your forearms instead of your hands. Your body should form a straight line from your shoulders to your ankles. Tighten your abs intensely. Hold for 30 seconds. Progress gradually to 45 seconds, then 60 seconds.

Side Bend, for your external and internal obliques: Stand with your feet hip-width apart. Place your hands together over your head. Reach toward the ceiling. At maximum height, start bending laterally to the left. Pause briefly in the stretched position and reach with your arms and hands, this time maximally to the left. Return slowly to the top center position. Do not let your hands move forward. Keep them extended and directly over your head. Reach toward the ceiling with both hands and repeat bending to the left side for the required repetitions. Rest for a few seconds with your arms hanging at your sides. Then perform the movement to your right side in a similar manner for the same number of repetitions.

Here's the order I'd recommend in a workout for the body weight exercises:

1. Calf Raise
2. Squat
3. Hip Raise
4. Wall Squat
5. Pushup
6. Crossed-Arm Crunch
7. Plank
8. Side Bend

I would suggest performing these exercises in a normal manner, one set of each for 8 to 12 reps, twice a week. After six weeks, you might want to try the barbell/dumbbell/machine workouts that are described in chapter 23.

Bonus Challenge!
Hey Buddy, Can You Spare a Couple of Weeks?

Question: Can you achieve really good results from only 2 weeks of the 6-week program?

In one of my recent groups of twenty women, I repeated the measurements and photos after the initial 14 days, then again after 42 days. I wanted to compare the overall averages at the end of two weeks and again after 6 weeks. Usually I do the before-and-after measurements and photos only at the start and end of the program.

But I thought: What's possible in only 2 weeks? Could you see some major differences in photos after 14 days?

Answer: Absolutely. Even a 1-pound muscle gain can make a difference in the appearance of a body part and how the surrounding fat and skin hangs. And a 5-pound fat loss is noticeable on most women.

The woman who lost the most was Katie Smith, who dropped 14 pounds of fat and is pictured in chapter 7.

In case you're curious, the all-time record for fat loss in 2 weeks for men in my program is 19 pounds. This individual was 6' 7" tall and weighed 302 pounds at the start.

On the following five pages are some individuals whose results after 2 weeks were among the best. I believe you will see that, yes, if you can spare a couple of weeks, then some major improvements are going to come into sharp focus.

Remember, the before-and-after comparisons in this section were taken 2 weeks apart. Two weeks is hardly enough time to see your hair grow, but it is enough time to better your body.

Why don't you make a commitment today and get started tomorrow? Two weeks will turn you into a believer.

Pam Waters

Age 60, Height 5' ¼"

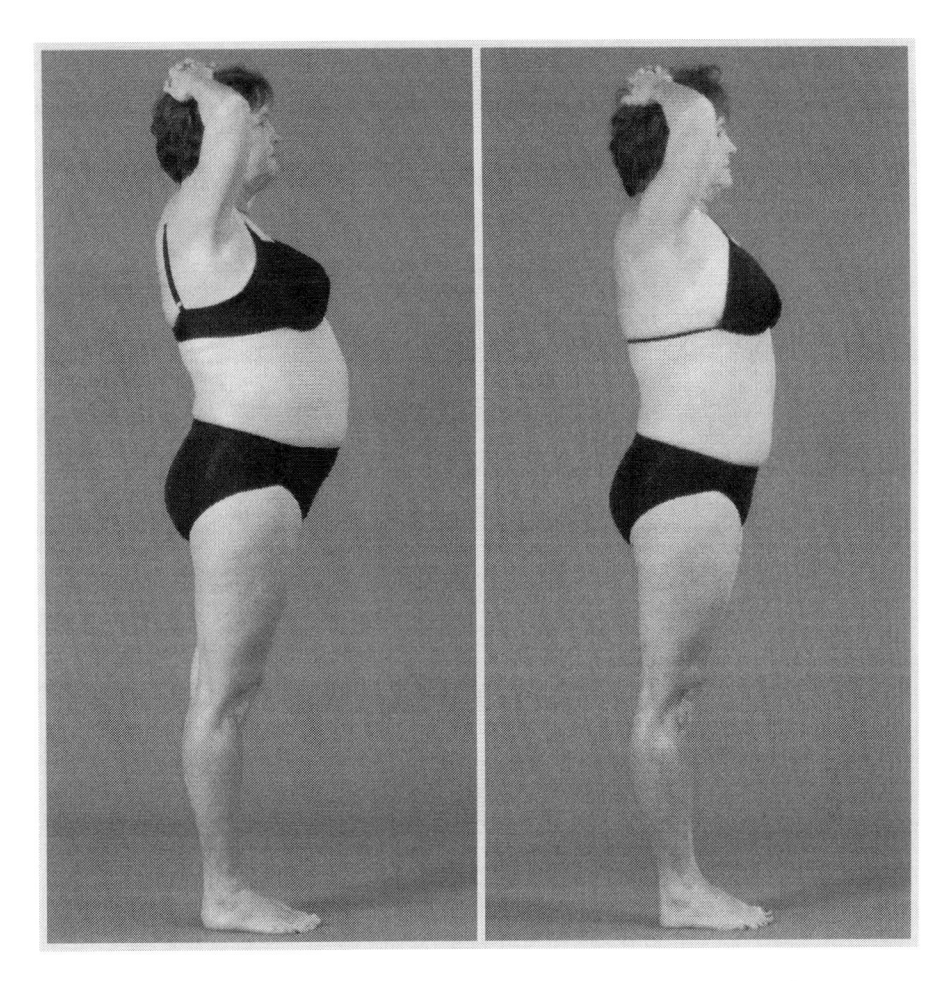

145.5 Pounds   **136.1** pounds

After 2 weeks
11.61 pounds of fat loss
3 inches off waist
2.16 pounds of muscle gain

"My stomach muscles during the exercises seem to be signaling my belly fat to go away. I didn't think that was possible, but it sure was happening to me."

Amy Barber

Age 48, Height 5' 6"

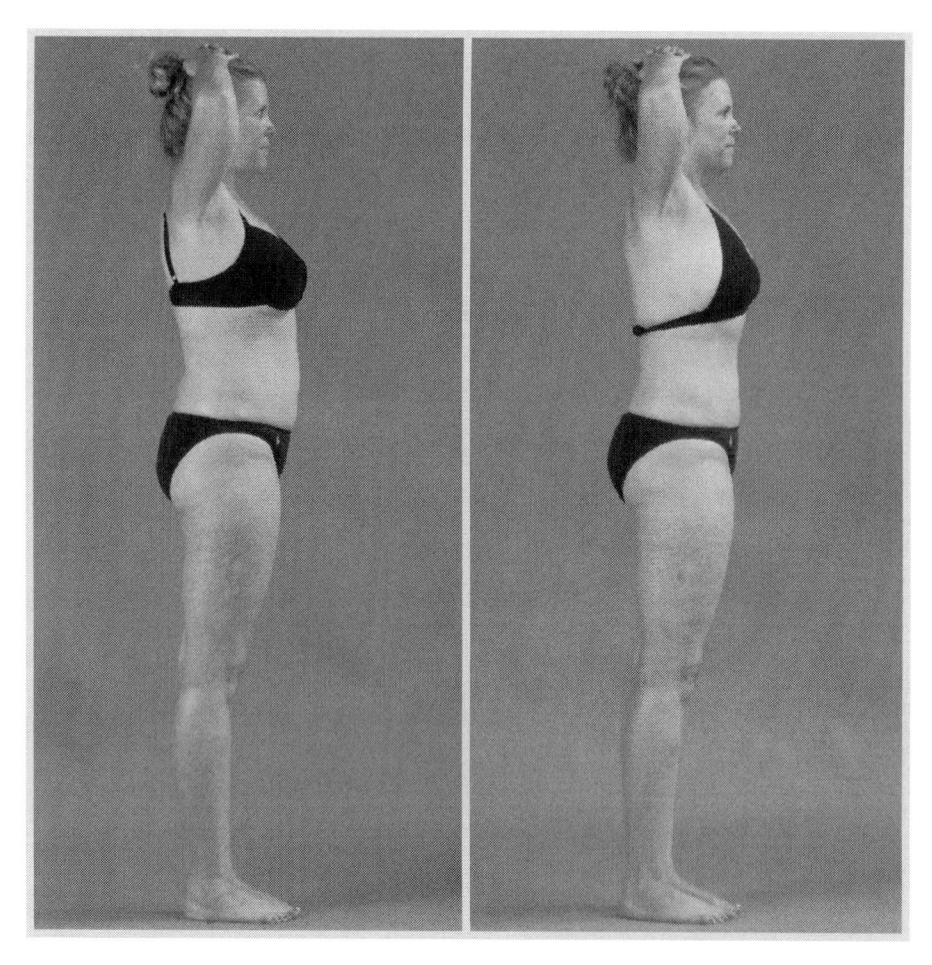

156.7 pounds   **146.1** pounds

After 2 Weeks
12.6 pounds fat loss
2.625 inches off waist
2 pounds of muscle gain

"Each day I'm on the move. Weeks 1 and 2 forced me to prepare. And preparation works. I have three kids and they are so proud of me and my results."

Nanette Carnes

Age 79, Height 5' 8"

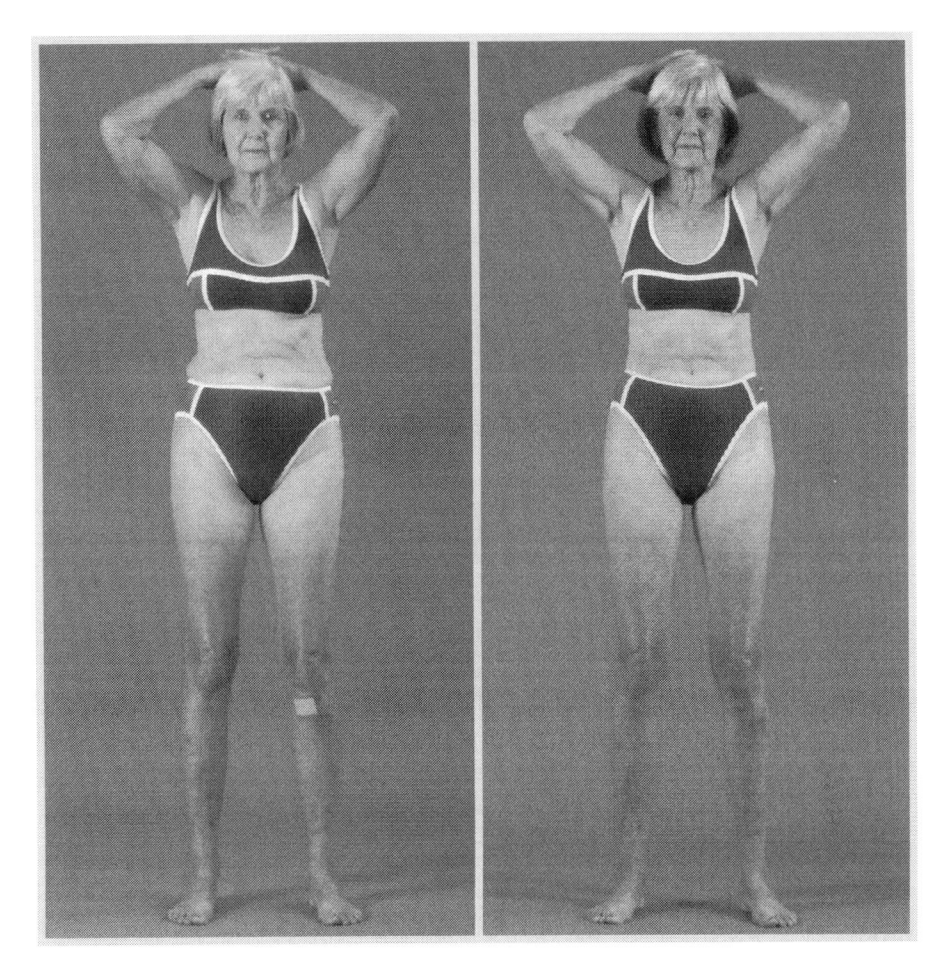

131.7 pounds   **120.4** pounds

After 2 Weeks
12.48 pounds fat loss
3.5 inches off waist
1.18 pounds of muscle gain

"For much of my life, I was a physical education teacher and remained active. Recently I've put on some fat around my waist. This program got rid of it and I'm pleased. Dr. Darden said I was the oldest woman he's worked with in Gainesville. I hope my results inspire other women my age to become involved."

Yu Yang

Age 46, Height 5′ 7½″

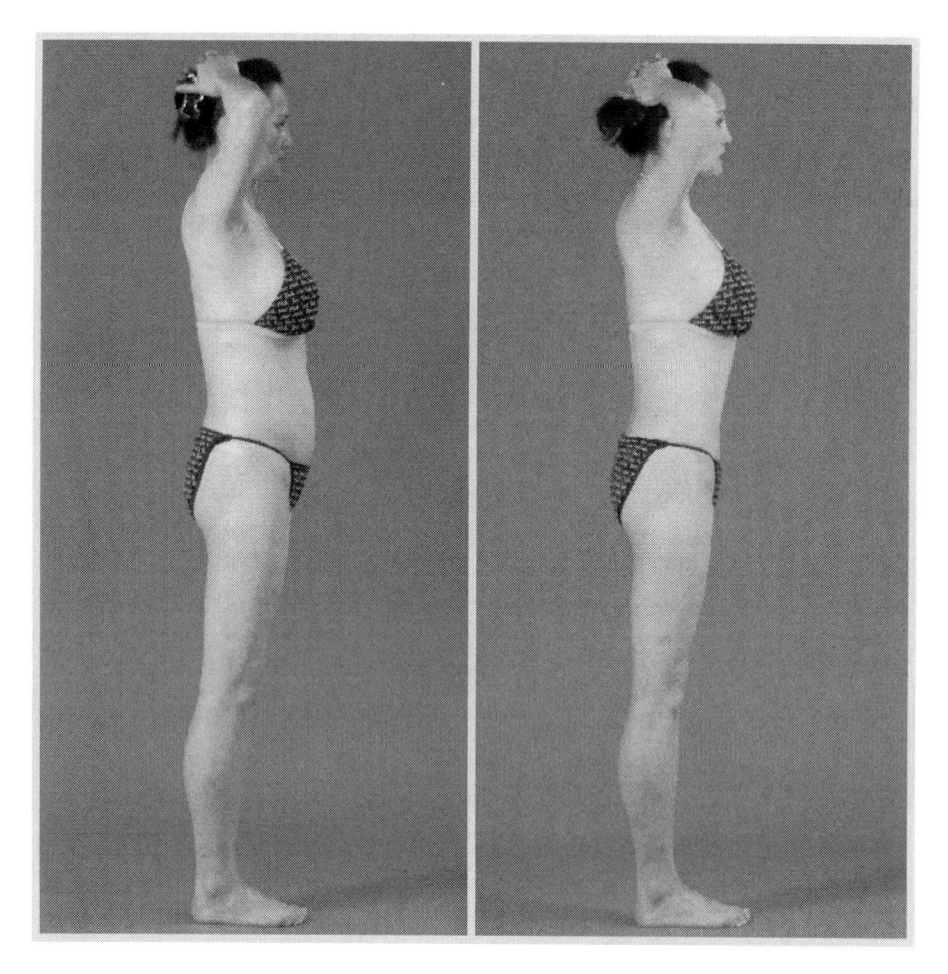

137.9 pounds   **128.9** pounds

After 2 weeks
10.3 pounds of fat loss
3.625 inches off waist
1.3 pounds of muscle gain

"The eating and exercising plan made me feel powerful . . . and I like that feeling."

Kristi Taylor

Age 39, Height 5′ 7½″

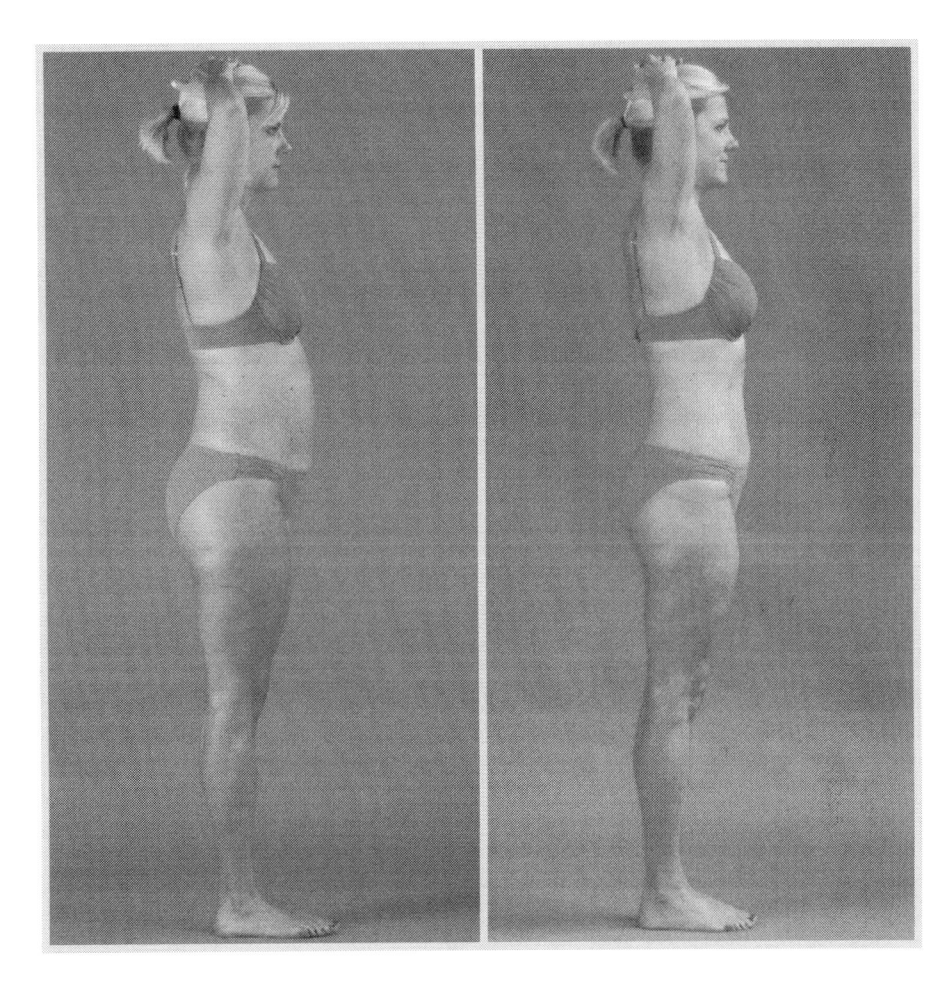

150.8 pounds   **142** pounds

After 2 weeks
11.4 pounds of fat loss
3 inches off waist
2.5 pounds of muscle gain

"I don't like the slow negative exercise. But it sure does work. My body responded quickly. My husband and our three kids have noticed a difference in my overall shape."

V

REJUVENATING YOUR LIFE

25 Still Living Longer Stronger

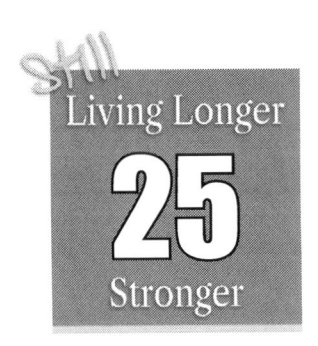

Improving Your Results

Maybe you lost 10, 15, or even 20 pounds of fat on the six-week course, but you've still got more pounds and inches to lose. It took you longer than six weeks to put it on—try twenty years—and it's going to take a little more time to get it off.

You probably have to weigh well over 250 pounds to lose 35 pounds of fat or more in six weeks. Yes, Angel Rodriguez, whom you met in chapter 2, removed 38 pounds. But Angel weighed 280 pounds when he started, and he was an exceptional individual. So, if you weigh less than 250 pounds and have more than 30 pounds of fat to eliminate, there's a high probability that it's going to require longer than six weeks. If you're in this category, here's what to do.

Make Another Commitment

Decide now that you want to continue. You've already taken some major steps toward removing your excess body fat. You've made significant progress by sticking with the plan for six weeks. Make a commitment for another six weeks—or less, if you believe you can reach your goal sooner.

Some people repeat the program three or four times—for a total of 18 to 24 weeks—before they reach their satisfaction level. Simply turn the week-by-week dieting, exercising, and other practices into week-by-week steps that move you closer and closer to your goal.

Take a Week Off

You may think I'm contradicting myself if I tell you to take a week off after I just asked you to commit to more diet and exercise. Most people who continue with the plan find that a week off renews their enthusiasm.

If you want to take a week off, be careful not to gorge yourself with food. You probably would have difficulty doing so even if you tried. Simply eat approximately 400–500 more calories per day than you were eating during Weeks 5 and 6, or approximately 1,500-1,800 calories a day. Keep drinking your water: 1 gallon a day.

After a week off, you'll be amazed at how eager you are to repeat the six-week course.

Repeat the Diet

Six weeks ago, in two-week phases, you gradually decreased your calories from 1,500 per day to 1,400 and then 1,300. Now that you've added a few pounds of muscle to your body, you should be able to progress through the same descending-calorie plan with similar results.

Furthermore, this time around you'll be more familiar with the menus and foods. You'll be able to gauge serving sizes without weighing and measuring. The entire process will be easier. Just be sure your daily calories remain at the appropriate level.

You may be wondering why this down-up-down plan is preferable to sticking to the same number of calories each day, week, and month. The down-up-down method is effective for three reasons:

- Such a diet supplies you with needed variety.
- A degree of irregularity seems to benefit the body's fat-burning process.
- When your calories go up, so does your energy level. Such an increase in energy level may be just the motivation you need to train harder and thus stimulate additional muscle growth.

You can continue this down-up-down eating plan for as long as six months, or until you attain your fat-loss goal.

Continue Your Strength Training

During the last two weeks of the six-week program, you did one set of eight exercises during each of your training sessions. You should continue with this routine of eight exercises two times per week until you lose your excess fat. Don't do more than eight exercises per session.

Your strength training goal is to double your strength in all your basic exercises. If you did 40 pounds for 10-10-10 on the biceps curl when you started, for example, then your goal is to perform 80 pounds for 10-10-10.

Austin Deely

Age 44, Height 5' 8"

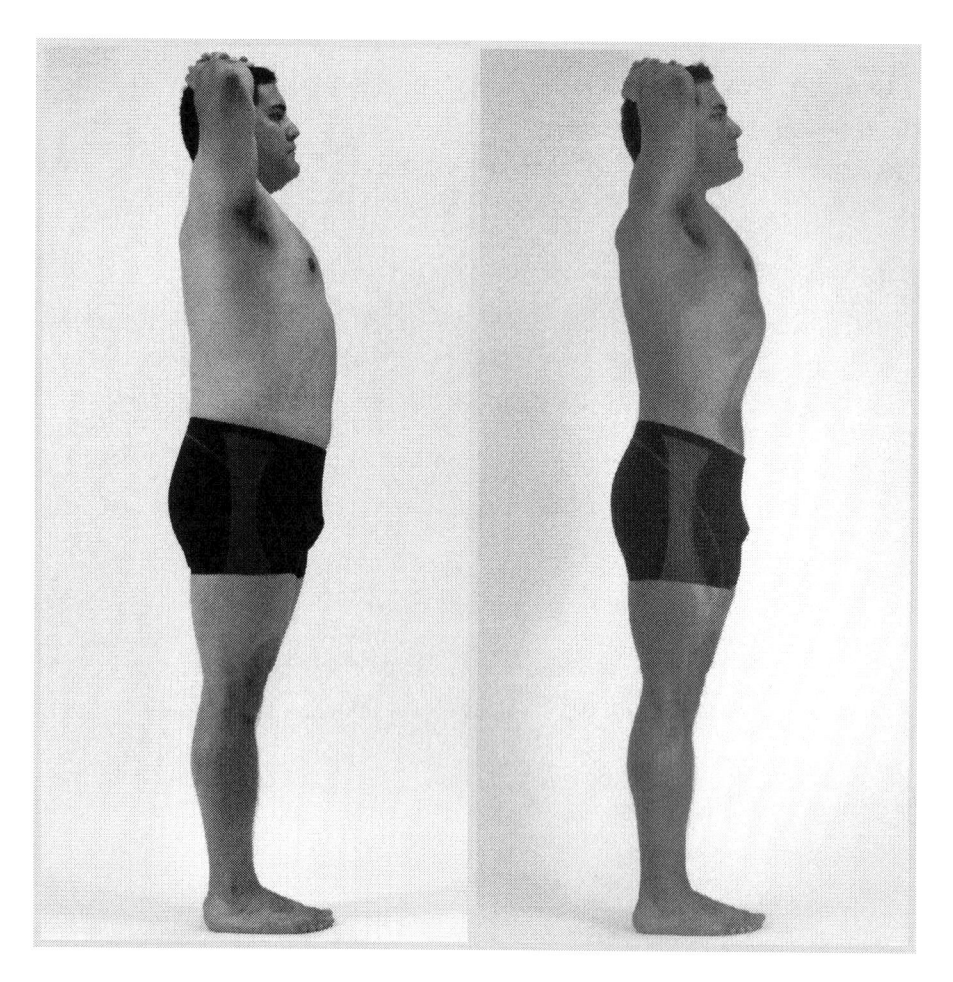

222.5 pounds   **185.5** pounds

After 12 Weeks
43.5 pounds of fat loss, **7** inches off waist
6.5 pounds of muscle gain

"I've wanted a muscular body for as long as I can remember. But I couldn't cut back on my calories for more than a couple of days. Dr. Darden's program taught me how to eat, manage, and achieve my goal."

Many people can reach that goal within four to six months on all their basic exercises.

Once this goal is reached, you should read and apply chapter 27 to your workouts.

Your other practices—such as water drinking, walking, and extra sleeping—should remain unchanged from Weeks 5 and 6.

Concentrate One Day at a Time

Patience is truly a virtue when it comes to losing those last few pounds of fat.

Hang in there. Those fat cells can shrink. Your dream, if it is realistic, can be accomplished. It does take time, however.

Be patient. Stick to the plan in this book. Take it one day at a time.

Make intelligent action your ally.

Still Living Longer 26 Stronger

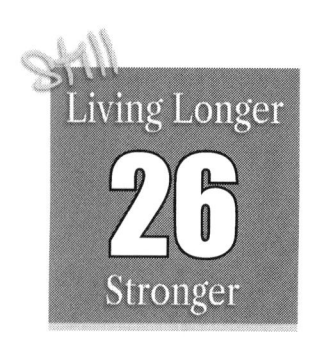

Maintenance Guidelines

Once you become satisfied with the condition of your body—whether it took six weeks, twelve weeks, or more—your next task is to maintain that status. Doing so requires certain adjustments to the guidelines and practices that you've been using up to this point.

Study carefully the following adjustments.

Adhere to a Carbohydrate-Rich, Moderate-Calorie Eating Plan

Your eating plan is still carbohydrate-rich, but you do not need to decrease the calories. Your calories are now raised to a moderate level. Instead of eating from 1,300 to 1,500 calories a day, you'll be consuming from 1,800 to 2,400 calories per day. Maybe you can even eat more after your new body weight has stabilized.

There is no simple way to determine in advance how many calories you will need to maintain your new body weight. Trial-and-error experimentation will make the level obvious, however.

You should probably begin with 1,800 calories per day and see what happens after a week. If your body weight keeps going down, raise the calories to 1,900 or 2,000, depending on how much weight you lost during the last week. Soon, you should reach a level where your body weight stabilizes. That level is your daily calorie requirement.

Always keep your calories rich in carbohydrates. The 50:25:25 ratio of carbohydrates, proteins, and fats is not only ideal for losing fat, but it is also appropriate for maintenance. Fruits, vegetables, breads, and cereals are your primary sources of carbohydrates. On your maintenance eating plan, strive each day to consume four to six servings of fruits and vegetables and four to six servings of breads and cereals. Doing so will usually allow your other foods, meats and dairy products to fall into correct ratio naturally.

Eat Smaller Meals More Frequently

You've been limiting your five meals per day to 400–500 calories or less. To maintain your body weight, set the limit per meal to 600 calories or less. A 600-calorie meal will keep your insulin responses small. Furthermore, 600-calorie meals are something you can easily adapt to most of the time.

What happens when you occasionally eat more than 600 calories at one time? Don't panic. Simply understand that you will sometimes backslide.

Anticipate, plan, and get back on track.

Drink 128 Ounces of Cold Water Each Day

I hope by now you've seen and felt the benefits of drinking plenty of cold water each day. Make it a permanent part of your new lifestyle to consume at least 128 ounces or one gallon of cold water per day.

Perform Strength Training Twice a Week

You never outgrow your need for larger, stronger muscles. As you age, larger and stronger muscles become more and more important. In fact, that's the theme of this entire book. Bigger muscles improve performance, add shape, stabilize joints, burn more calories, and consequently allow you to live longer stronger.

Remember, as your muscles get stronger, you need less total exercise.

Walk After Your Evening Meal

Walking on a full stomach is a great way to relax and burn extra calories.

Although you may not feel it's necessary to walk every day of the week during your maintenance plan, you should still take advantage of the benefits of walking.

Sleep an Extra Hour Each Night

Extra sleep is like extra water: you didn't know what you were missing until you tried it. It will be to your advantage to maintain your new sleeping schedule every night you can.

Avoid Overstress

Some medical authorities believe that overstress is the real culprit behind obesity, high blood pressure, heart disease, the divorce rate, and just about everything else that plagues today's aging men and women. Certainly, too much stress can seriously limit your body's ability to lose fat. And too much stress can ruin your maintenance plan and cause a return to your old ways of coping. Don't let this happen to you.

Stay calm and stay in control.

Fight Disinformation With Facts

Disinformation is especially prevalent on the Internet. In 2013, someone on Twitter trying to reinforce a point noted a quote purportedly from Albert Einstein: "If the facts don't fit the theory, change the facts."

That is certainly a thought-provoking statement from a famous scientist such as Einstein. Except Einstein never said that. Few people noticed the mistake, and that untruth was circulated and recirculated for years.

Einstein was a believer in facts and rules, which he used to combat disinformation. It took him two decades to test, retest, and finally confirm the theory of relativity. Would Einstein, in a moment of haste, ever have changed facts to support his theory? Absolutely not.

The Maintenance Guidelines in this chapter are based on sound facts and rules—facts and rules that lead to bigger muscles, leaner bodies, and more productive lifestyles. *Still Living Longer Stronger* took me more than half my life to finalize. The facts utilized within help me daily . . . and they will help you, too.

Apply facts. Fight disinformation. Maintain basics.

27 Still Living Longer Stronger

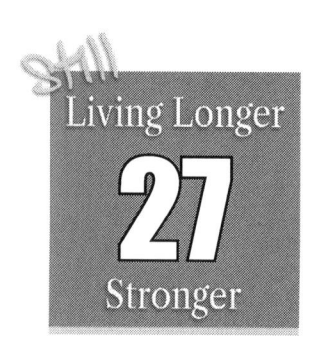

Advanced Strength Training Techniques and Workouts

In my hardcore training books—such as *Super High-Intensity Bodybuilding*, *Massive Muscle in 10 Weeks*, and *The New High Intensity Training*—I teach readers more than a dozen advanced techniques. Some of their names are *pre-exhaustion*, *double pre-exhaustion*, *stage reps*, *hyper reps*, and *negative-only*. These books and techniques, however, are designed for experienced athletes who are under the age of 40.

Still Living Longer Stronger is for men and women over the age of 50. In fact, some are in their 70s, 80s, and 90s. Thus, there is only one advanced technique in this chapter, and it is called 30-10-30.

But be forewarned: 30-10-30 is an intense method that will challenge you.

30-10-30

For six weeks, you've used the 10-10-10 method, which is a 10-second negative followed by 10 regular reps and a finishing negative of 10 seconds. The 30-10-30 advanced technique triples the negative time of both negative phases. In other words, it involves two 30-second negatives with 10 regular reps in between. Instead of the set being over in 50 seconds, it now requires 90 seconds—which makes it significantly harder and more advanced.

The following is an example of doing a biceps curl using this advanced technique.

30-10-30 Biceps Curl With a Barbell

Similar to 10-10-10, the 30-10-30 technique for the standing biceps curl is best performed with the help of a training partner who has a watch with a second hand. Begin with a resistance on the barbell that is 10 percent less than what you'd normally do for your 10-10-10 set. Have your training partner assist you in getting the initial repetition into the top position.

Begin the slow lowering, as your training partner calls out the seconds: 5, 10, 15, 20, 25, 30. Try to be halfway down, where your forearms are parallel to the floor, at the 15-second mark. Breathe and continue to move slowly.

At the bottom of the 30-second negative, switch to doing 10 faster positive/ negative repetitions. Take about 1 second on each positive and 2 seconds on each negative movement.

After your last positive repetition, do a finishing 30-second negative with the same 5-second guides. Note: If you've selected the resistance correctly, that final 30-second lowering will be very difficult.

Don't be surprised if you must sit down after this 90-second set. A minute or so later, you should feel a pronounced pump in your biceps muscles—which is good.

With a little preparation, the exercises that you've used in your 10-10-10 workouts may be adapted to the 30-10-30 technique.

Remember to breathe freely as you perform each 30-second lowering. Do not hold your breath or grit your teeth.

30-10-30 Exercises

The exercises with a shorter range of movement—such as the calf raise, the shoulder shrug, and the abdominal curl—do not work well for the 30-10-30 style. Too much of the range must be held motionless as opposed to gradually moving. Here's a list of the single-joint and multiple-joint exercises I recommend for use with 30-10-30:

30-10-30 Single-Joint Exercises

    Leg Extension on Machine
    Leg Curl on Machine
    Biceps Curl With Barbell
    Hammer Curl With Dumbbells
    Triceps Extension With One Dumbbell

30-10-30 Multiple-Joint Exercises

    Squat With Dumbbells
    Squat With Barbell
    Leg Press on Machine
    Pulldown on Lat Machine
    Overhead Press With Barbell
    Bench Press With Barbell
    Bent-over Rowing With Barbell

30-10-30 Workouts

I've organized a series of workouts for 30-10-30. Generally, because of the intensity of 30-10-30, a workout requires only six exercises, while the frequency remains at twice a week.

Below is a listing of these advanced workouts.

Advanced Workout 1

    1. Squat With Dumbbells
    2. Bench Press With Barbell
    3. Bent-over Row With Barbell
    4. Overhead Press With Barbell
    5. Biceps Curl With Barbell
    6. Triceps Extension With One Dumbbell

Advanced Workout 2

    1. Squat With Barbell
    2. Bent-over Row With Barbell
    3. Triceps Extension With One Dumbbell
    4. Hammer Curl With Dumbbells

5. Bench Press With Barbell
6. Pulldown on Lat Machine

Advanced Workout 3

1. Leg Curl or Leg Extension on Machine
2. Leg Press on Machine
3. Overhead Press With Barbell
4. Bent-over Row With Barbell
5. Triceps Extension With One Dumbbell
6. Biceps Curl With Barbell

The recommended way to start the three Advanced Workouts is as follows:

- Perform Advanced Workout 1 twice a week for two weeks.
- Perform Advanced Workout 2 twice a week for the next two weeks.
- Perform Advanced Workout 3 twice a week for the following two weeks.

After that six-week period, you can mix the workouts on your own.

28 Still Living Longer Stronger

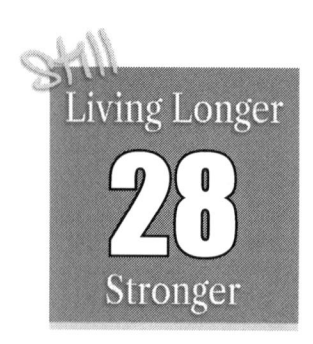

"I Feel Twenty Years Younger!"

"My body was a mess," Marlene Hill remembered. "And I was in the gym five times a week, doing yoga, Pilates, Zumba, and spin classes as well as the sauna and hot tub. But none of it seemed to reduce my body weight.

"I tried various diets, including Weight Watchers, but I only dropped a few pounds on each, and what I'd lost always came right back. I was 59 years old and the scale was still climbing. I felt depressed all over."

Marlene decided it was time for a change.

"When I heard Dr. Darden at an introductory meeting discussing the differences between *weight* and *fat*," Marlene continued, "I realized I had been confused by the terms. I had spent so much time working on the wrong things and not enough focusing on real concerns: fat and muscle."

The first time I saw Marlene, I knew she would be great for my Still-Living-Stronger-Longer program. I could tell she cared about her health and appearance.

"I have a lot of belly and torso fat," she noted seriously. "When I was 21 and living in Caracas, Venezuela, I was into modeling. My body was much different then. I was lean and angular. I've had two kids, who are adults now, and I'm divorced. I want my modeling look again."

My challenge to Marlene was as follows: "To get your decades-ago shape back, you've got to quit shutting your body down with too much activity. You must rethink the basics: work harder on your muscles, eat the right foods, and drink lots of water. No more sauna and hot-tub baths. These guidelines, performed seriously, will shrink your fat cells and forge new muscle."

Marlene, with a determined look, announced: "I have a dream that I want to achieve—and I'll follow your plan in detail, I promise." And wow, did she ever.

In six weeks, Marlene removed 20.12 pounds of fat and 4 inches off her waist, while adding 3.17 pounds of muscle to her arms and legs.

"My dream shape has returned," Marlene said, smiling, "and I feel twenty years younger."

Marlene Hill

Age 59, Height 5' 6"

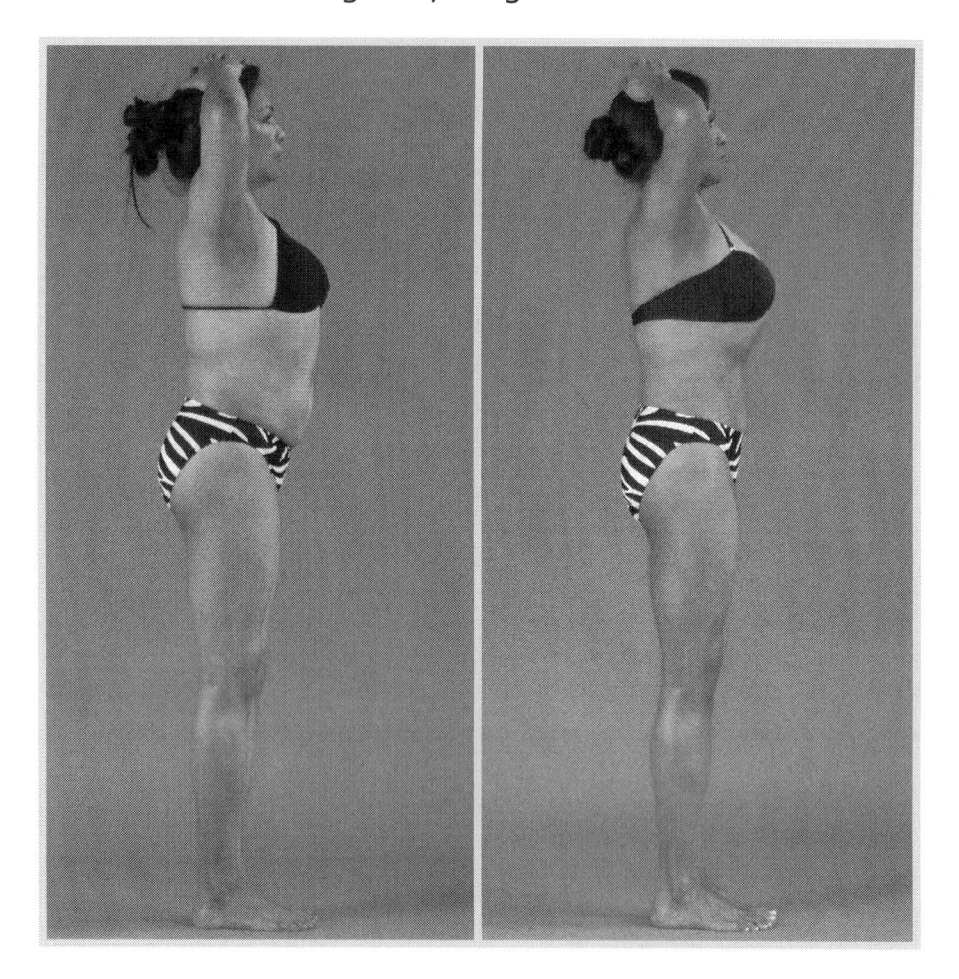

157.7 pounds   **140.75** pounds

After 6 Weeks
20.12 pounds of fat loss
4 inches off waist, **4** inches off thighs
3.17 pounds of muscle gain

"I'm so happy that my belly has shrunk. Now I feel much more alive and sexy."

Living Longer 29 Stronger *(Still Stronger)*

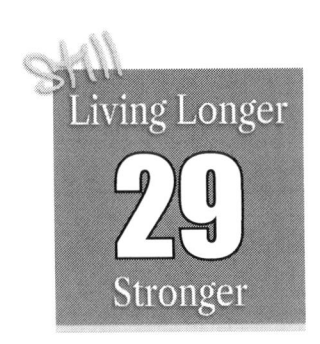

Dancing on Your Troubles

Concluding chapters are often difficult to write because you want your reader to be both challenged and inspired. Of course, there also needs to be a connection with the theme of the overall book.

The part titles throughout this book begin with the prefix "Re–": Resolving, Reexamining, Rebuilding, Reducing, and Rejuvenating. By now you know that all this reworking of actions and processes is crucial. This chapter touches those bases in a meaningful way. But some unexpected surprises will surface also.

A *Northern Exposure* Story

An old friend recently loaned me his DVD collection of *Northern Exposure*, the popular CBS-TV drama series from the early 1990s.

The setting of the series is a small town in Alaska called Cicely, and the main characters are a young doctor (Joel Fleishman), a beautiful woman who is a bush pilot (Maggie O'Connell), and interesting people who reside in and around the town. *Northern Exposure* is one of my all-time favorite TV shows.

An inspiring episode from season 3 involves Ruth-Anne Miller—an elderly woman who runs the general store—and her young assistant, Ed Chigliak. Ruth-Anne has a matriarchal role in the community, and Ed, an orphan from a nearby indigenous tribe, is the sincere and helpful, but naïve and inexperienced, kid around town.

Ruth-Anne's 75th birthday is approaching, and Ed is very concerned about her advanced age and her health. She has broken a bone in her foot, and she must stay off it and keep it elevated for several weeks. Ed is working overtime feeding and caring for her, and he's worried, especially since one of her best friends recently died at age 72. Ed decides, after careful observation and analysis, that he has to find the perfect birthday gift for Ruth-Anne.

The Perfect Gift

The town holds a birthday party for Ruth-Anne on Friday night. As the event ends, Ed pulls Ruth-Anne aside and unveils his gift, a heavy package the size of a shoebox.

Ruth-Anne unwraps the package and removes the lid. With a perplexed look on her face, she thanks Ed for the . . . "well, ah . . . dirt." The box is full of dirt. "What's it for?" she asks.

"It's extra-special dirt," replies Ed.

The scene changes. It's the next morning and Ed is leading a hobbling Ruth-Anne, with a single crutch, up the side of a nearby mountain.

"Where are we going, Ed?" Ruth-Anne asks, almost out of breath.

"This is the spot . . . right here," says Ed with a satisfied look on his face as he kicks the dust off his boots.

A Beautiful Mountain View

"Oh, Ed, the view is beautiful," says Ruth-Anne as she looks out over a majestic tree-lined valley to even higher peaks. "But why did you walk me up here?"

Ed points down at Ruth-Anne's feet. "Because this is the exact location. This is where you will soon rest."

Ruth-Anne still doesn't know what Ed is implying.

"Ruth-Anne," Ed says, "the special dirt in the box last night came from this spot. It was a part of my birthday present to you. I bought you this small plot of land. When you're buried here, you can look out over this beautiful valley and mountains. You'll never ever feel lonely in these surroundings."

Suddenly Ruth-Anne understands what Ed has been trying to tell her: he fears she will die soon and be lonely, and he wants her to be well prepared and laid to rest among the trees and mountains she loves.

Choosing her words carefully, she thanks him for the grave plot and says she sincerely appreciates his feelings.

Then she explains to him that she has recently had a thorough medical examination (which Ed mistook as a sign of a serious problem) and that she is healthy. She is not going to die anytime soon. But, if she does pass away, then that will be fine, too—because she has led a full life composed of work, hobbies, marriage, children, fun, and travel.

Ed, however, is still concerned, especially since Ruth-Anne has been in such a subdued, reflective mood.

Sensing the overly serious mindset of the moment, Ruth-Anne looks at the young man and says, "Ed, there's one final birthday wish I have."

One Last Wish

"What's that?" Ed replies.

"I want us both . . . to dance on my grave."

Ruth-Anne throws her crutch to the side and starts dancing on her burial plot to an upbeat tempo. As the camera pans back, Ed starts to smile. Ruth-Anne laughs. Ed laughs. And Ed joins her in the dancing.

Then the camera moves to an aerial view and looks down on Ruth-Anne and Ed dancing faster and faster as the dust starts to rise. The music gets louder as the camera pulls away, and Ruth-Anne and Ed gradually blend into the dust, rocks, trees, and mountains. They all become one—or, as Carl Sagan and Stephen Hawking might say, "One with the Universe."

Wow, I thought to myself as the credits rolled. *That was some great writing and acting—and what a thought-provoking ending.*

My Gift to You

My gift to you is not a gravesite but a *lean, strong body with solid brain power,* which will keep you healthy and out of the cemetery for many decades.

To keep your transformed body *permanently* lean and strong, you must have the discipline to follow the guidelines in this book not just for 6 weeks or 12 weeks, but for the rest of your life.

Look often at the before-and-after pictures in this book, and reread the stories of the individuals who have successfully applied the SLLS program. Each one has beaten the odds with discipline and gained an above-average amount of muscle. Don't forget, muscle adds fire, action, and life to your metabolism.

Appreciate often that *Still Living Longer Stronger* is based on science.

Appreciate, too, that life demands before it rewards. You must *do* before you can *have*. When you're tough on yourself, life becomes more purposeful, more productive, and—ultimately—less demanding.

The rules that I've challenged you with in this book are seldom glamorous and sometimes hard to face. But practicing these guidelines, as you have done, leads eventually to the lifestyle changes that must occur for year-after-year permanence.

Hang Smart

In your quest for a long life full of health and happiness, the next time you must make a difficult choice, I want you to remember the story of Ed and Ruth-Anne.

Celebrate facing tomorrow by dancing on your troubles today.

Dance, Relax, Enjoy

For much of my life, I have been described as *seriously serious*. Now, at 80 years of age, I believe it's time to welcome some less-than-serious dancing.

May we dance, relax, dance, and enjoy *Still* Living Longer Stronger.

30

Living Longer *Still* Stronger

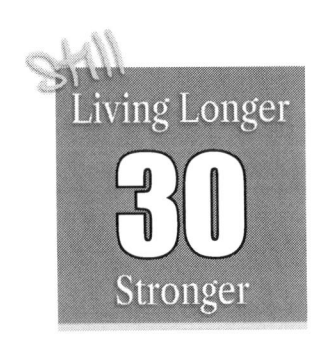

It's Still Working

You've got to be motivated and focused to keep your lost fat off. According to research, three years of maintenance is a valued signpost that you've conquered your fatness, and five years is even better.

This chapter features four men and five women who have done exactly that, and more.

I've known many of the people in this chapter for more than twenty years. I worked with Kirk Wilder and Blake Boyd in Dallas, Texas, in 1987. And I trained Peter Fleck and Jane Knuth in Orlando, Florida, in 2000. All of them were successful in losing fat and, more importantly, keeping that lost fat off.

Some of my trainees, unfortunately, have regained the fat they originally lost. I want each of them to know that you are still on my team . . . and I want to help you get back in shape. Please get in touch with me. You are always welcome in any of my courses.

But this chapter is about celebrating some folks who have beaten the odds. Each one has taken the long-ignored physiological principle of *building muscle to lose fat* and fully incorporated it into their lifestyles.

It was exciting for me to be part of a system that helped over-fat and out-of-shape men and women remold their bodies in ways that improved their appearance and are now letting them live longer stronger.

The names in this chapter have not been changed. These subjects freely allowed me to use their photographs, measurements, and interviews.

These are real people—just like you and your neighbors—who have jobs, spouses, kids, pains, problems, and highs and lows, just like you do. They've pushed through them all and managed to not only survive but thrive.

Yes, *Living Longer Stronger* worked for these men and women. And it's still working. Long after the headlined year, each person has remained lean and strong.

It Worked for Me in 1987

I lost 12 pounds of fat quickly, returned to my 34-inch waist, and have kept it off for thirty-six years. It's amazing the success you can have when you follow proven science instead of the latest fad. I'm 78 years old.

KIRK D. WILDER

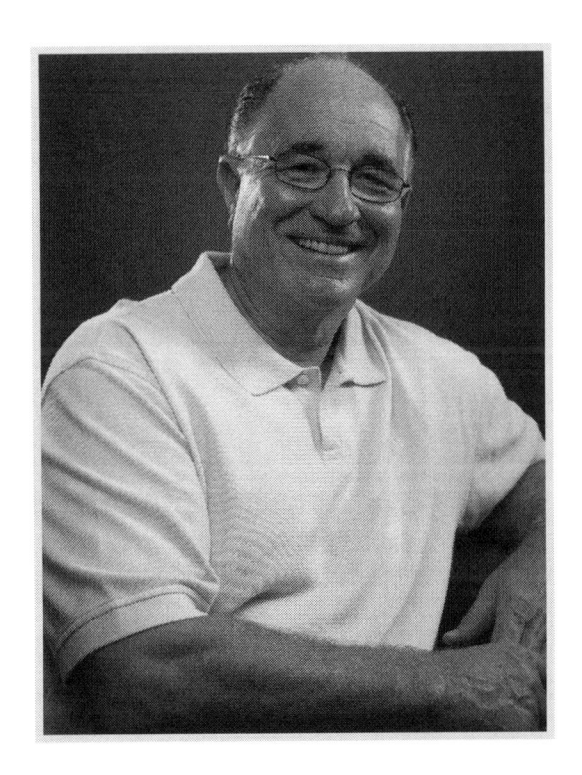

I'm the past president of Utopia Food and Fitness in Dallas, Texas. Our company was struggling in 1987 to find a credible weight-loss program that not only worked but lasted. Dr. Ellington Darden had a system that he said offered 100-percent fat reduction, plus muscle gain.

In 1990, we had UT Southwestern Medical Center test the plan completely.

Southwestern proved that a participant using Dr. Darden's program could, in fact, shrink significant fat, enhance lean muscle, and increase metabolism.

We know just about everyone in the fat-reduction industry, and Dr. Ellington Darden and his program stand at the top of our list, far above the others.

It Worked for Me in 1988

Going through Dr. Darden's program, and being on the cover of his book *The Nautilus Book* (1990) helped launch my career as an actor in Hollywood.

BLAKE BOYD

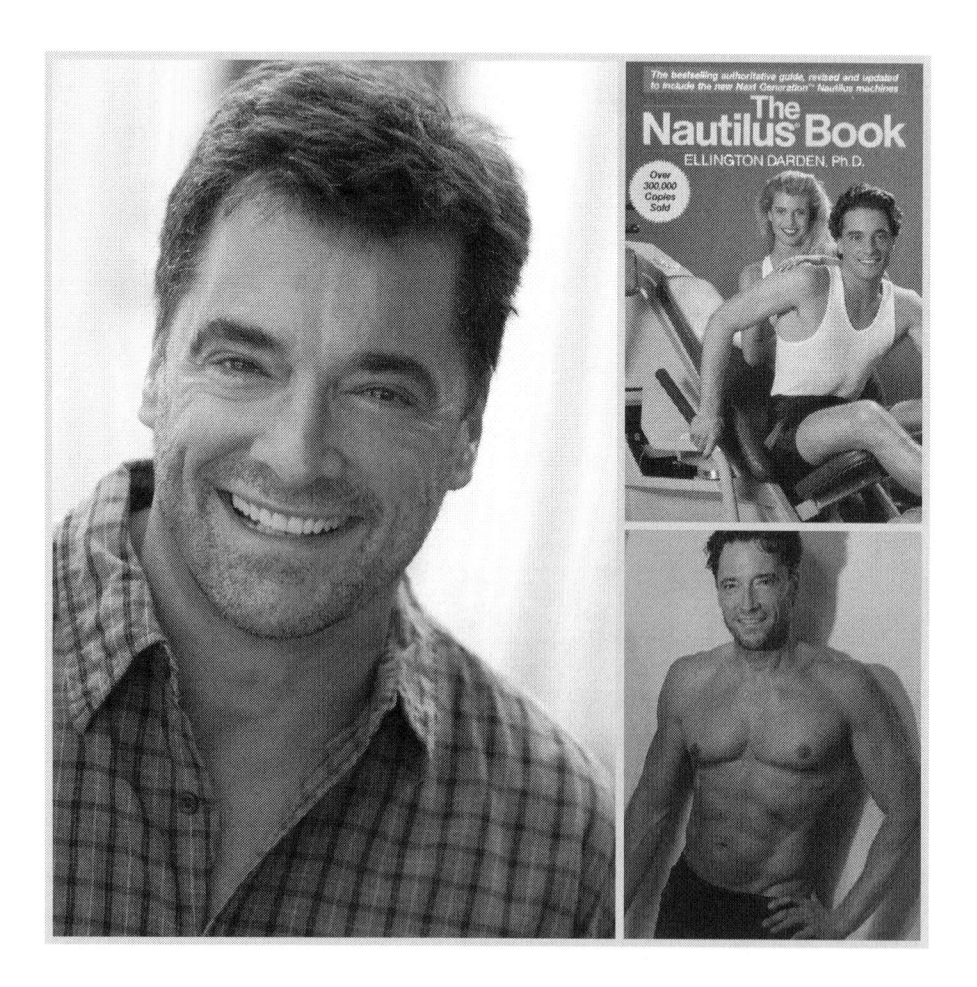

Blake Boyd, age 57, has acting credits in eighty productions, including the films *Out of Time* and *Cash Collectors* and the TV shows *General Hospital*, *Shameless,* and *Second Chances*.

He also has had roles in theatre in Los Angeles and New York.

It Worked for Me in 1991

I challenged myself at Gainesville Health & Fitness in the 1990s and got into the best shape of my life. My two teenage sons told me recently, "You're the most fit mom of any of our friends." At age 58, I'm nearly ten years older than any of the other moms, so it is quite the compliment.

JILL BITTNER

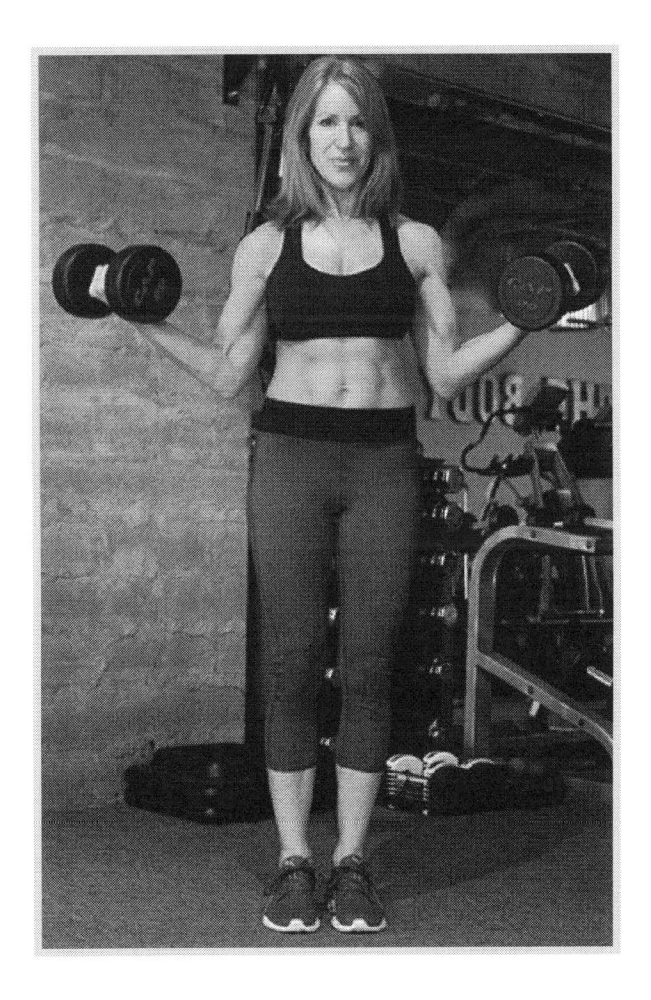

Jill finished my *Two Weeks to a Tighter Tummy* program in 1991 with 13.6 percent body fat, which is an excellent level. She has almost the same percentage today as she did then—and she's a lot stronger.

It Worked for Me in 2000

I lost 24 pounds of fat in 6 weeks and 4.25 inches off my waist and have kept them off for twenty years.

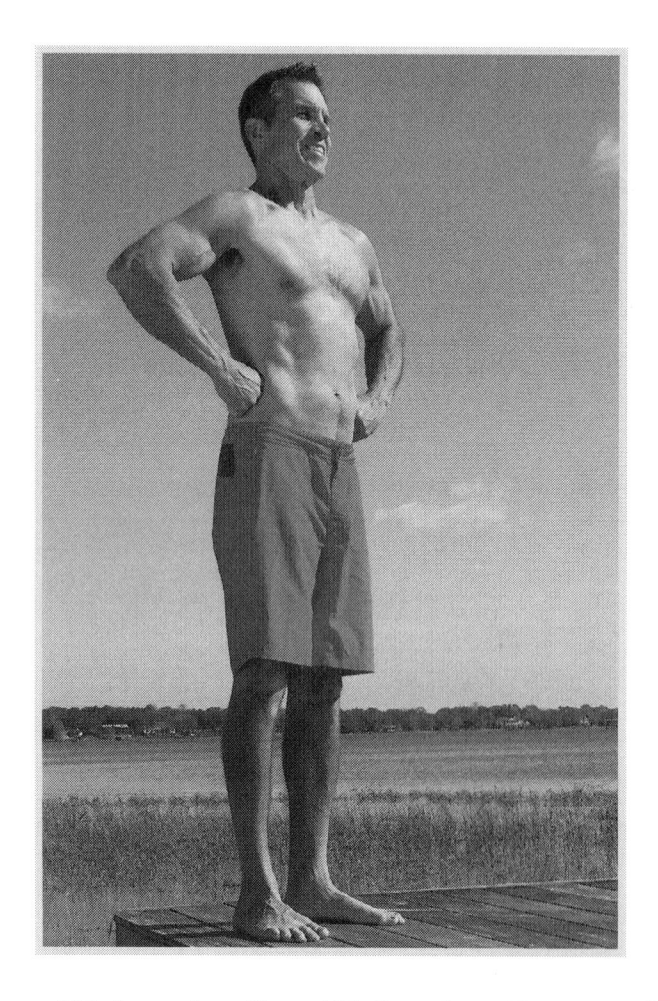

PETER FLECK

Peter Fleck, age 57, is a nine-time US Barefoot Figure Eight Champion. He's an active member of the Waterski Hall of Fame.

It Worked for Me in 2000

After marriage and two kids, I had 20 pounds that needed to come off. I did Dr. Darden's program in 2000, and in 6 weeks my extra fat was gone. Twenty-three years have passed. Anytime my body weight goes up 2 pounds, I use what I learned back then to get them off quickly.

JANE KNUTH

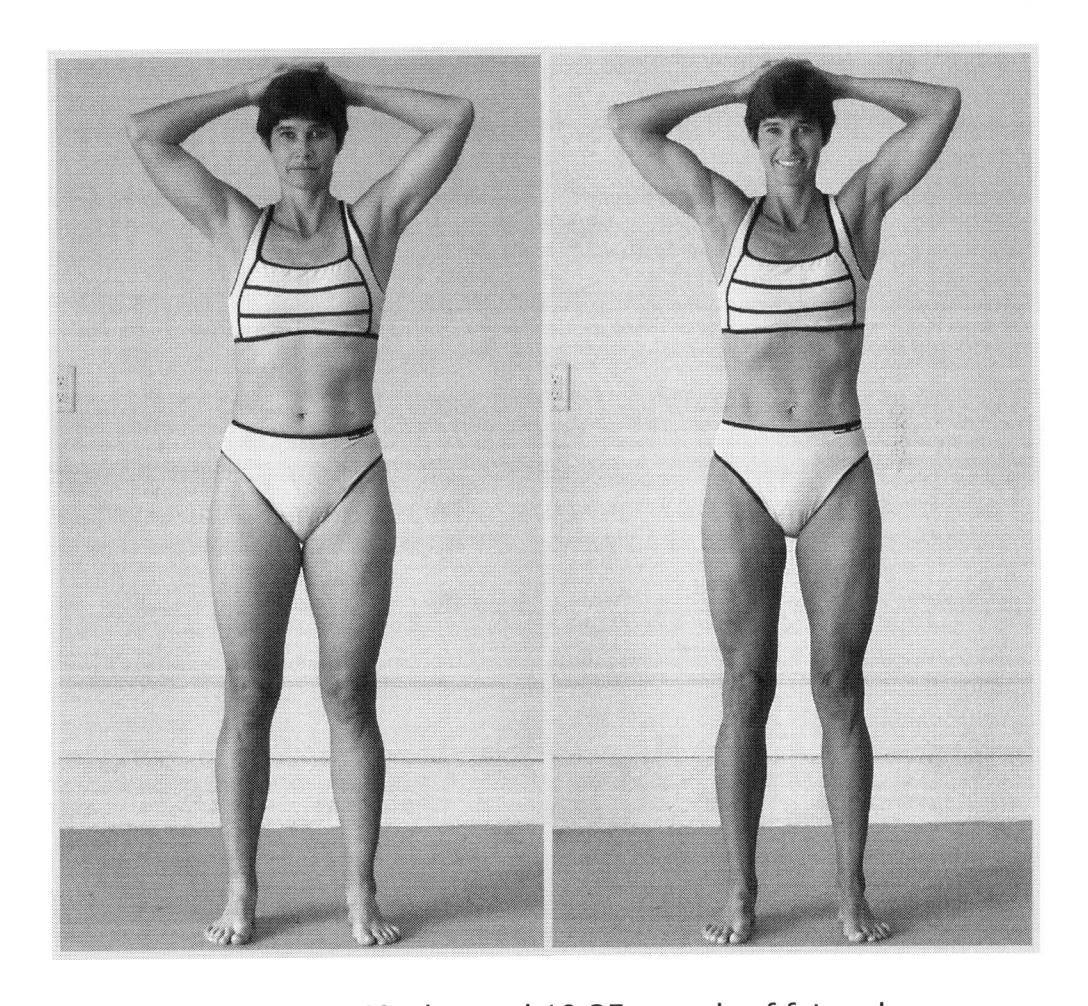

Jane, age 40, dropped 19.25 pounds of fat and 4.25 inches off her thighs in six weeks.

It Worked for Me in 2008

I've tried many diets, and Dr. Darden's is by far the best. I dropped 30 pounds of fat and removed 6 inches off my waist.

MAX MEDARY, MD

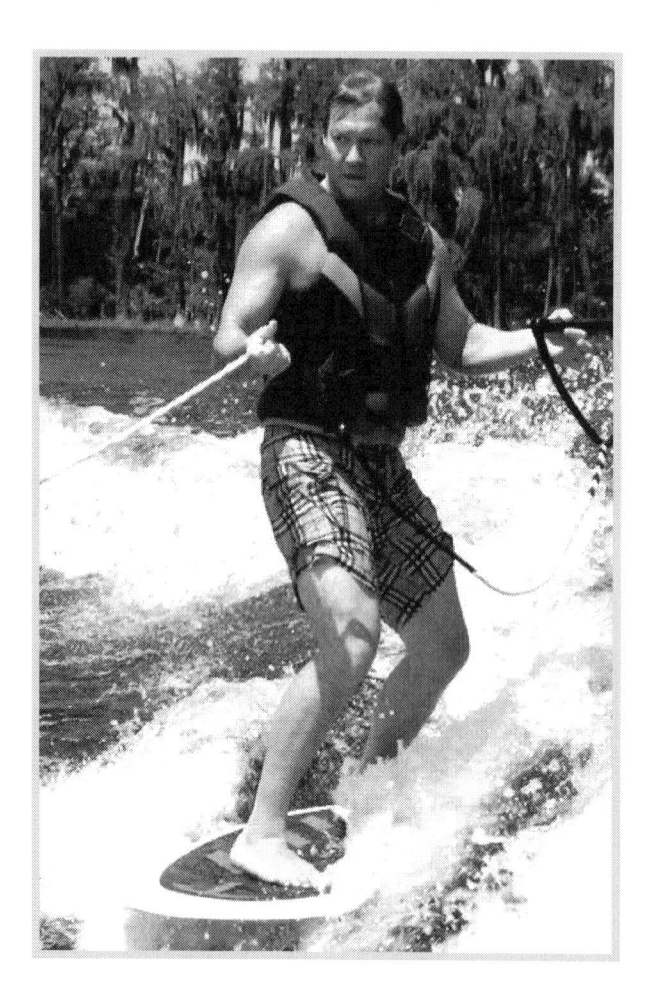

Dr. Max Medary is a 59-year-old neurosurgeon in Orlando.

Besides dropping significant fat, he built more than 11 pounds of muscle. He knows firsthand the importance of big, strong muscles and solid brain power.

Dr. Medary is an active sportsman in water sports, ice hockey, and lacrosse.

It Worked for Me in 2009

You've got to push yourself, or be pushed, to get those last reps. You've got to make yourself get more rest and sleep. Then, your growing muscles will help shrink your fat.

ROXANNE ACHONG-COAN, OD

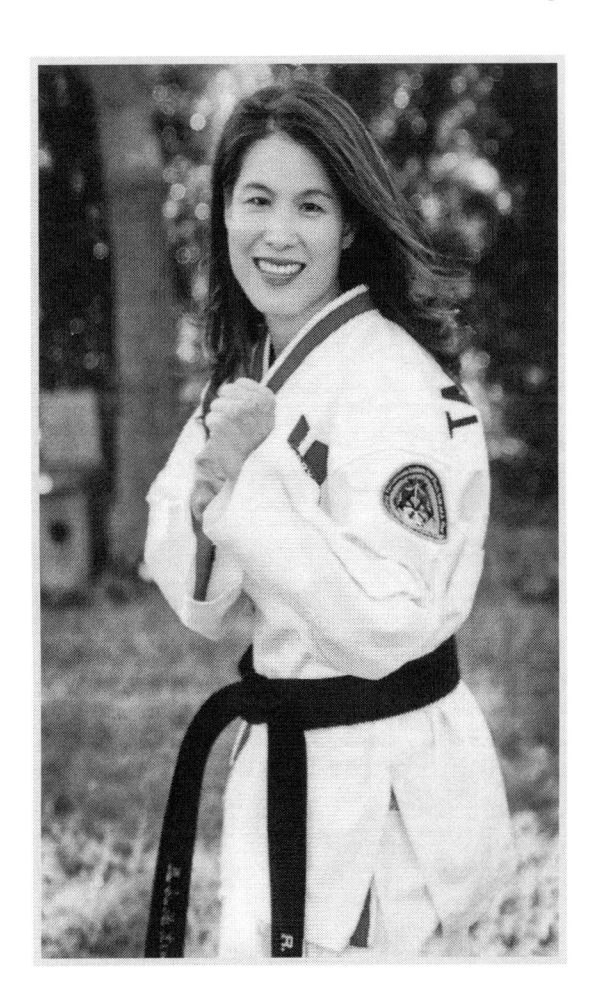

Dr. Roxanne Achong-Coan, age 51, experienced a body transformation.

In 2009, she built 8.4 pounds of muscle to help her lose 17.4 pounds of fat.

She practices optometry with her husband, Mark, in Ocoee, Florida.

She is also enthusiastic about martial arts.

It Worked for Me in 2010

I trained with Ellington Darden for three months and lost 9.25 pounds of fat and built 7 pounds of muscle. His principles have helped me keep my body at 138 pounds—for the last thirteen years.

TERRIE ATKIN

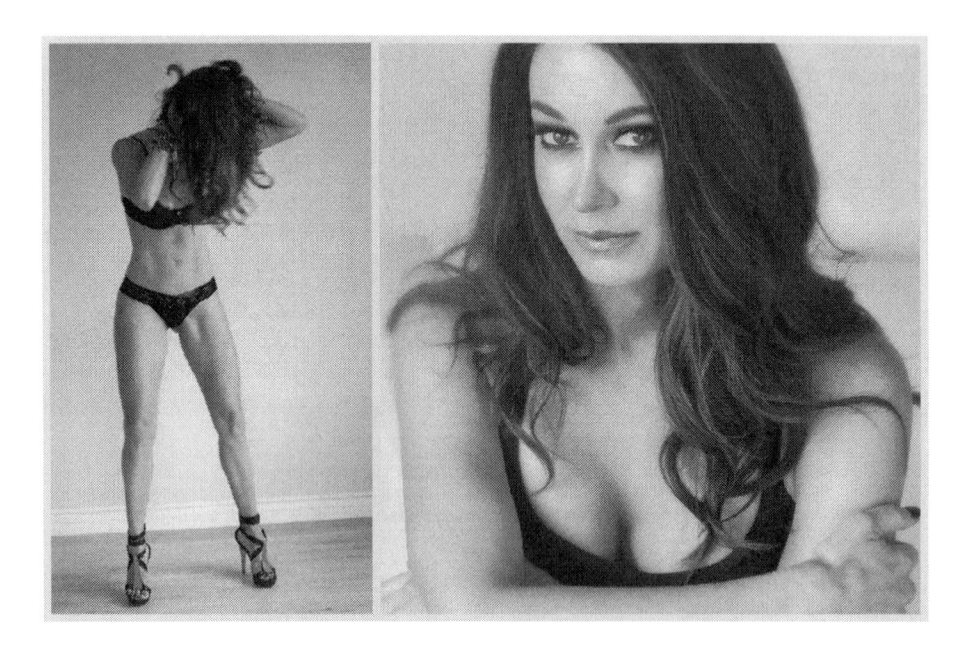

Terrie Atkin and her family lived across the street from the Dardens in Windermere, Florida, for a year. Then they lived in California for six years before finally moving to Bend, Oregon. At age 50, Terrie is 5' 9", with 14 percent body fat. At one time Terrie was a critical care nurse. These sexy photos of her were a gift for her husband, Ray.

Ray's critical care is now *sizzling*.

It Worked for Me in 2010

Back in 2010, my husband, Keelan, and I signed up for Ellington Darden's personal coaching. His training involved the practice of the primary requirements involved in this book. The course was tough, but doable. Over 12 weeks, Keelan lost 31 pounds of fat and built 4 pounds of muscle. My body weight went down 15 pounds and my strength almost doubled on the basic exercises.

BARBIE PARHAM

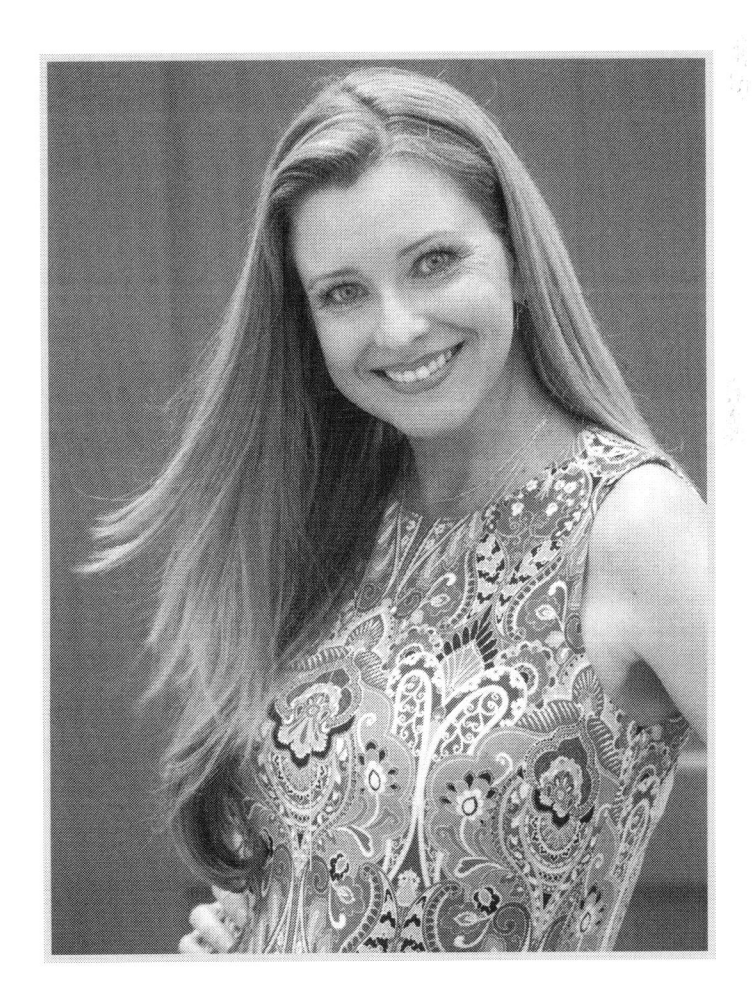

I'm now 50 and I've kept my 135-pound body stable for thirteen years and counting. I still train with Ell once a week.

Now, It's Your Turn to Experience

Still Living Longer Stronger

It Will Work and Keep Working for You

VI

RETELLING LOST STORIES: MEMOIRS

A Jog Down Memory Lane

In the fall of 1994, several months before *Living Longer Stronger* was published, I was talking on the phone with John Duff, the book's editor at Perigee in New York. John had great flair with his edits and always had suggestions that were timely and on target.

I was disappointed that he had red-flagged one of the last chapters of the manuscript. "It's not that I don't like the writing," John said, "because it's full of personality. But, Ellington, the place for this piece is in your memoirs."

John was correct. *Still Living Longer Stronger* is in many ways part of my memoirs. So I've selected six articles that were published more than two decades ago at Classic X, my first website, and I'm including them here as Part VI, chapters 31 through 36.

"Mirror Shine," the title of chapter 31, was also the title of the chapter that John Duff omitted. It's all about shining shoes to a high luster. Chapter 31 is dedicated to my mother and father, Barbara Lamar and George Bybee Darden, and my dad's parents, Sallie Dougherty Bybee and Thomas Ellington Darden. Each one understood the *why* of shined shoes and how they could open many doors.

"Do You Have Change For a Dollar?" (chapter 32) is about a laundromat across the street from Gainesville Health & Fitness and some of the characters I met there.

"Wanted: Dead or Alive" (chapter 33) begins with a dramatic Arthur Jones story from New Year's Eve, 1995. It ends with a group of influencers.

Of all the pieces I've researched and written in my lifetime (and there must be 400 or more), "Good Vibrations" (chapter 34) got the most attention. More than twenty-four years after the article was first posted, I still get email comments about it. That means it is still being circulated.

The next selection, "The Rest of Your Life" (chapter 35), was composed in 2000 and is my quest to get my audience to read—yes, read—more.

Chapter 36, "The Transition of Knowledge," is incredibly special and it has been a focal point for me over the last twenty-five years of my life. Transitions build bonds.

Settle into an easy chair with a cold drink, and get ready for the retelling of some of my favorite stories.

Still Living Longer 31 Stronger

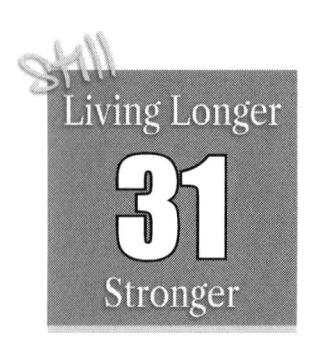

Mirror Shine

In the 1980s, I frequently lectured on strength training to high school coaches who attended the MacGregor Coaching Clinics, which Nautilus Sports/Medical Industries co-sponsored for many years.

During one of the basketball clinics in Chicago, I was in the walkway near the back of the auditorium eating a continental breakfast and visiting with a few friends. Several well-known coaches were speaking before my presentation, and I was sizing up the setting. Many coaches were passing by, grabbing a quick snack, and moving into the lecture hall. After a while, I felt a tap on my shoulder.

"Excuse me, but I'd like to shake your hand," a deep voice said. I wiped the last drink of orange juice off my mouth, pitched the napkin aside, turned around, and shook the huge hand of an elegantly dressed man.

"I couldn't help noticing your shoes," he continued. "I've always taken considerable pride in mine—the shinier the better—and you've got me beat. I want to compare notes, but right now I've got to get up front."

He quickly rushed away, and I never got a chance to say anything other than . . . thank you.

That big man in an olive-green, double-breasted tailored suit, with shoes almost as shiny as mine, was Chuck Daly.

At that time, he was the head coach of the NBA's World-Champion Detroit Pistons and was the next presenter. Since I was due in front of the group immediately after Coach Daly, I never got a chance to follow up with him. But I did visit with one of his assistants. He said Daly was obsessive about his shoes, that he had dozens of pairs and kept them all brightly polished. "Sometimes, I think he'd rather talk about shining shoes," smiled the assistant coach, "than shooting basketballs."

I would've certainly liked talking shoes and shines with Chuck Daly—and perhaps some hoops, too.

Readers over the age of 60 will have an interest in shining shoes. Why? Because we grew up doing it daily, or certainly weekly. Even you guys in your 40s, or anyone in the armed forces, will identify with many things I'm going to cover.

My interest in shining shoes started with my grandfather.

My Grandfather's Shoes

I don't remember much about my grandfather. He passed away when I was 5 years old. His name was Thomas Ellington Darden, and his friends called him Ell, as they did me when I was growing up.

One thing I do remember about him was his black cap-toe shoes, which were manufactured by Stacy Adams. These dress shoes, when he shined them, sparkled like oil on water. In the right light they looked like a black mirror.

After my grandfather died, I spent a lot of time visiting with my grandmother. She would babysit my sister and me on most Saturday nights, while my mother and father played bridge with friends. Between the typical coloring, drawing, learning to play dominoes, and making fudge, we often talked about him.

Grandfather was not a wealthy man. He owned a grocery and dry goods store in Willis, Texas, a small town eight miles north of Conroe, where I was raised. Grandma said he liked to buy a new suit and a new pair of shoes every spring, until the Great Depression hit. Then, he had to make do with what he had for more than ten years. He compensated by keeping his shoes highly polished.

He loved to fiddle with his shoes, she said, and he did so every night while we listened to the radio. Some Saturday nights, Grandma would bring out Grandpa's shoes—along with brushes, rags, and polish—and I'd practice polishing them, with her help.

When I was in the sixth grade, Grandma gave me a shoeshine box, with all the trimmings, for my birthday. Wow, I was excited. I got out my oxfords and polished them that night.

I still remember my grandma saying: "Shoes are the most important part of dressing for a man, and he better keep them shined."

That box, besides containing all the brushes and polishes, had a foot-rest on top. It wasn't long before I felt like I was confident enough to walk downtown and shine shoes on the corner for 10 cents. On a good Saturday I might shine the shoes of a dozen men. The best part wasn't the money—it wasn't that much—it was observing the men as they walked away. Every single one of them walked taller and acted more confidently. Furthermore, shiny shoes, for some reason, make you smile more.

High School Contests

When I entered high school in 1959, the style of dress for boys was a sport shirt, blue jeans, white socks, and loafers. I had two pairs of loafers: black and cordovan. I took pride in keeping them polished. Before school most mornings, all the guys who polished their shoes would compare their shines in one area of the school grounds. It quickly became no contest, as I always won. My shoes were the only ones with a mirror finish.

The mirror finish was sometimes called a spit-shine because it required a special technique of combining wax polish and the exactly right amount of moisture. Once you have built up enough of a base shine, then you can brighten it quickly with a dab of wax and saliva—hence the term spit-shine.

Often one buddy, David Pyle, who could come close to my shine, accused me of putting sole dressing on the toes of my shoes. Sole dressing was an enamel that was painted on the edges and heels of the shoes. It was put on last to add the finishing touches to the shine. Putting it on the toes of the shoes would make them shine more, but it would easily chip and mess up the leather.

Sole dressing on the toes was considered cheating. I'm sure some of the scratches I found on the toes of my shoes after football and basketball practices were put there by David Pyle, as he just couldn't believe that my shoes weren't covered with sole dressing. They weren't!

Sometimes after practice I'd find gum on and in my shoes. That just spurred me to make my shoes better than ever the next day.

Ever since I graduated from high school in 1962, I've kept my best shoes brightly shined. Granted, in Florida, I don't wear my highly polished dress shoes often. Sandals are on my feet most of the time. But when I wear a coat and tie, I always take out my good shoes and touch them up before I put them on.

The Best Shoes

If you want an extraordinary shine, you've got to have a quality pair of leather shoes with smooth, fine-grained leather on the toes and anywhere else you want a polished look. The best shoes seem to come from England. The English shoes are heavier, finer grained, and more carefully assembled.

I've traveled to London several times, and the shoes I've purchased there are superb.

My best dress shoes are made by Alan McAfee. You can buy them in the United States at Church's Shoe Stores. I have a favorite pair of cordovan loafers that I can get a great shine on by using oxblood polish. I purchased them in a small shop in London named Foster & Son.

I know some of you like Italian-made shoes. Their soft leathers and workmanship make them a comfort to wear, but I've never been able to get a high-gloss shine from the softer, thinner Italian shoes.

American-made shoes vary greatly. Most of the time, however, you get what you pay for. The higher-priced dress shoes do seem to take a better shine. Today, Allen-Edmonds makes a fine cap-toe shoe for the businessman.

As far as color goes, black shines best. I've never been able to get a superior shine out of any brown or tan shoes. If I wear brown, I choose a suede finish, which requires brushing, not shining. Cordovan, however, is a horse of a different color. This burgundy color can be shined to a degree that, for whatever reason, may equal black.

The Best Polish

Although there are many polishes available, the one I believe is a cut above the rest is Kiwi. Kiwi's paste wax is unsurpassed. In fact, "Parade Gloss," the version sold in England, which has recently been introduced into the United States, is my personal favorite. Those British guards with the shiny black boots and tall headdresses, who surround the Queen's London palace, use this polish. You must try it.

I'm also partial to Kiwi saddle soap, brushes, sole dressing, and other shoe accessories.

The Mirror Shine

Here's the step-by-step procedure—passed down from my grandfather—that I've used for seventy years to yield a shine that's as reflective as a mirror.

1. Use shoe trees inside your shoes to stretch the leather to the natural shape of your feet. Keep the trees in your shoes when you shine them.

2. Wipe any noticeable dust or dirt off your shoes and soles with a damp towel. Always do this with a towel and never your shoe brush. Cleaning your shoes with your brush will get dirt in the bristles. This dirt may be transferred back to your shoes during the shining process, which involves some brushing. Dirt, if you don't already know it, is the enemy of a shine. That's why it's important to clean your shoes properly before you polish them.

3. Lather up some saddle soap and brush it on the tops, sides, and bottoms of your shoes. Yes, I said bottoms. Cleaning the soles of your shoes not only preserves them better, but it keeps the potential dirt farther away from the tops and sides.

4. Wipe off the saddle soap softly and carefully. Your shoes should now be squeaky clean.

5. Find a well-lit area to do your polishing. A desk next to a window works best, as you'll get the benefit of natural lighting.

6. Cut a piece of smooth cotton cloth approximately 2 inches by 4 inches. An old cotton tee shirt will suffice. Cut the cloth in half so you have two 2-inch by 2-inch pieces. Wrap the piece of cloth around a small cotton ball. This cloth around the cotton ball is what you're going to use to apply the polish to the shoe. You'll use the second cloth and another cotton ball later. Also, you need a small saucer and an ice cube. Take your shoes, polish, brushes, cloth, cotton balls, and ice cube to the well-lit area and sit at a desk or table.

7. Open the can of paste-wax polish. Take the cloth-surrounded cotton ball and dampen it slightly on the ice cube. Cool water facilitates the spreading and drying of the paste wax on the leather. Rub the cloth on the wax and spread the polish on the shoe in small circles. The idea is to use only a moderate amount of wax each time. I start in the middle at the tongue of the shoe, move down to the toe, and then cover the sides. I repeat the same procedure on the other shoe. Both shoes now have a dull appearance from the unbuffed wax. Pick up the first waxed shoe with one hand and the soft brush in the other.

8. Brush the shoe smoothly with long strokes. Repeat with the other shoe. Examine each shoe closely and touch up with polish any dull or rough area. Buff it out with the brush. For a higher gloss, use a shine cloth next.

9. Fold the shine cloth until it's about the size of your wallet. Sprinkle some of the ice water across the tops of each shoe and vigorously polish with the cloth. Give special attention to the toes. The idea is to get them to shine as much as possible—before the most important steps. These last steps are what separate a good shine from a mirror shine, or what was commonly called a spit-shine. They involve taking the second cloth-covered cotton ball and slowly working a small amount of polish and cold water onto the shoe until even a brighter shine emerges.

10. Apply the polish in very small circular motions. Keep working on each area, which should be only the size of a quarter, until the shine comes through. A little cold water helps seal the wax. Too much water, or too much wax, however, will dull or water-spot the shine. You're better off having too little water and wax, rather than too much.

11. Continue polishing quarter-sized areas over your entire shoe. Again, give the toe area special attention. At first, you may think the shine will never come, but it will. Just be patient. The gratifying thing is that day after day, week after week, month after month, the shine keeps getting better and better. Finally, a true mirror finish emerges. In fact, it usually takes three or four weeks of almost daily shines to build a significant base. Once you build a significant base, your polishing time is reduced drastically.

12. Buff with a piece of nylon wrapped around your index finger in short strokes for even more sparkle. This is especially appropriate for those hard-to-get-at places around the seams, laces, and any area that needs consistency. The nylon can come from the toe of an old pair of socks or even pantyhose. Nylon, unlike cotton, doesn't absorb polish—so it does the best job of adding a final glow to the shine.

13. Edge your soles and heels with a light coat of sole dressing. Sole dressing can build up quickly, so it is only necessary to apply it once every five or six shines.

Follow these thirteen steps consistently for a few weeks and you'll soon have a mirror shine that will draw attention from anyone who appreciates shoes and style.

Parallels

There are parallels between shining shoes and strength training. They both require discipline and patience in building a base. Once you have a solid base, the process gets easier. Furthermore, highly polished shoes get attention, as do lean, strong bodies. Don't underestimate the importance of getting attention today.

I can still hear my grandmother relating that my grandfather thought you could tell a lot about a man by the shine of his shoes . . . and not just the shine on the toes, but also the backs and sides. Many businessmen in the 1930s, she said, built their wardrobes from the ground up: shoes before suits and shirts. "Highly shined shoes," Grandma said, "meant that the man was successful."

I remember a segment from the popular TV series *Matlock* where Andy Griffith, who plays the aging attorney, is shown in his office shining his shoes prior to presenting his final argument to the jury. "There's a dull spot right here on my right instep," Matlock motions to his assistant as he dips his cloth into the water and wax, "that just might convict my client. That jury will surnuff notice it if I don't polish it out."

I believe Matlock was correct. Juries do notice the shoes of attorneys. Little things do make a difference.

Frank Pacetta, author of *Don't Fire Them, Fire Them Up*, would agree with Matlock. Pacetta is credited with turning around Midwest sales teams at Xerox. One of his top ten sales tips is: Dress and groom yourself sharply. "I give brushes and cans of polish to reps who have trouble keeping their shoes shined," writes Pacetta. There's no room for the scuffy-loafer salesman on his team.

Besides the parallels above and the actual shine on the shoes, there was something else about the entire process that was meaningful to me.

Solitary Pleasures

I never completely understood why I liked to shine shoes, but I knew I did. Working with the hands on small, precise tasks always provided me a certain amount of satisfaction. At times it could be therapeutic.

I gave it little thought until I read *Maybe (Maybe Not)* by Robert Fulghum. Fulghum talks about how he gets great solitary pleasure out of ironing his own dress shirts. From the cuffs to the collars to the plackets, he details how he learned this skill from a housekeeper who watched over him when he was growing up. The ironing process was slow and deliberate. It couldn't be hurried. Fulghum's description made me think of my grandmother and how she helped me establish skill and pride in shining shoes.

Then Fulghum writes about how, years later, he journeyed to Japan to live in a Buddhist monastery. There, he was commanded to do mundane tasks to focus his mind. One day his job was to rake the gravel paths throughout the monastery gardens.

All morning and all afternoon he raked, and raked, and raked. Toward the end of the day, he had a sudden realization. Raking a gravel path right was just like ironing a shirt correctly. Adhering to the details with efficient precision, Fulghum noted, was the Buddhist doorway to understanding.

Simple, seemingly boring things—once you lock into the experience—can expand your mind to new levels.

At that moment, I knew what Fulghum was feeling. I had experienced the same thing many times as I shined my shoes—the solitary pleasure of the eye, hand, cloth, polish, and leather becoming one. You never, never hurry such a process. Rushing dulls the shine and clouds the mind.

I'm sure you've had some of these solitary pleasures. Weeding in the garden, detailing the car, chopping wood, painting the garage, and fishing with a cane pole—sometimes we use these times to reflect and talk to ourselves. Sometimes it even becomes active meditation.

Shining Longer Stronger

Whatever success or failure I've had at whatever else I've tried to do, deep down I hold this engraved fact:

> At the very least, I can shine shoes . . . shoes that would make my grandmother, grandfather, and even Chuck Daly proud . . . shoes that could put me into the Shoe-Shining Hall of Fame.

In the hustle of today's business environment, when I need solitary pleasure—I often shine my shoes.

Shoe shining is a part of my Still Living Longer Stronger.

Still Living Longer 32 Stronger

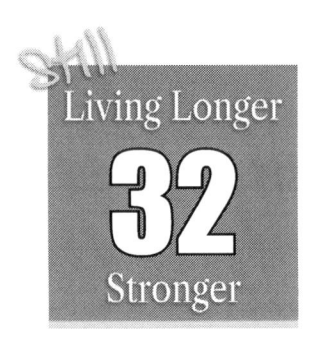

Do You Have Change for a Dollar?

Wednesday is laundry day for me. That's right, I do my own laundry—and I've done so for the last twenty-five years with my washer and dryer at home.

But when I lived a hundred miles north, in Gainesville, I visited a coin laundromat on University Avenue. There were some interesting things about that old laundromat that I really liked.

First, it was convenient. It was located between the Gainesville Health & Fitness Center, where I did research for my books, and my townhouse, which was only a two-block walk from the laundry building.

Second, it was in a small strip shopping center, which was a hub of activity. On one side was a Subway sandwich shop, a Handyway store, and a small post office. On the other side was a shoe store, a barber shop, and a video rental place. And across the street was the fitness center, which is the largest fitness club in the United States. It has 20,000 members, and 4,000 people train there on most weekdays.

Third, the woman who worked at the laundromat was a memorable person. Her name was Millie.

Millie's Specialty

When I first met Millie, she was 70 years old, stood 5 feet tall, and weighed 92 pounds. She had deep wrinkles over her face from too much sun and too many cigarettes. She was meek, soft-spoken, and—you could tell from her actions—a hard worker for much of her life.

Most of all, Millie knew washing and drying: backward, forward, inside, and out. "The key to getting your laundry right," Millie used to say, "is not overloading the washer, the correct amount of soap (less is best), a hot dryer, and quick fold."

What's quick fold? Quick fold, according to Millie, keeps the wrinkles out of most clothes. You remove clothes from the dryer immediately and you begin folding the ones you want the fewest wrinkles in: your best shirts and trousers first, for example, and your underwear and socks last. Her folding techniques, however, were implanted from decades and decades of experience.

Take tee shirts, for instance. Anyone who exercises owns dozens of tee shirts. If you're like me, you dislike wearing a tee shirt that's covered with wrinkles. But how do get the wrinkles out, especially if you don't like the thought of ironing a tee shirt? The secret is in the folding.

Quick Folding a Tee Shirt

Here's how Millie instructed me to fold a tee shirt:

1. Remove it from the dryer quickly and make sure it's right side out.

2. Hold the shoulder seams, one in each hand, and swish the entire tee shirt in front of you in big strokes through the air. Do the swish twice.

3. Spread the tee shirt flat on a table. The front should be face down with the shoulders farthest away from you.

4. You are now going to make two vertical folds on the shirt. Take the left sleeve and shoulder and fold it (left to right), from one-third to two-thirds of the way across and down the tee shirt. Smooth out any visible wrinkles with your hand.

5. Take the right sleeve and shoulder and fold it (right to left), from the two-thirds to the one-third division. The sleeves should now be neatly wrapped, one on top of the other, over the back of the shirt. Again, smooth out any wrinkles.

6. Grasp the bottom of the shirt and fold it in half horizontally. Smooth any wrinkles and fold the shirt again in half horizontally.

7. Turn the material over and you have a neat, folded, approximately 6" × 12" collar-up tee shirt—which will be virtually wrinkle-free when you unfold and wear it. It is now ready for storage in a drawer or basket.

Well, I'm telling you, Millie could fold a tee shirt faster than anyone on the planet. One morning I watched her fold twenty-five tee shirts in something like 3 minutes. I was so amazed that I timed her on the next one: **5 seconds flat**.

Since Millie's laundromat was located just down the street from the campus of the University of Florida, she dealt with thousands of students. She would do washing, drying, and folding at the rate of 50 cents per pound, or offer free advice if you wanted to do it yourself. I usually preferred to do it myself, especially since I enjoyed conversing with Millie.

Good-Bye, Millie

In 1996, at age 75, Millie retired. I kept using the facility until I left Gainesville eighteen months later, but it just wasn't the same without Millie. The man who owned the laundromat hired at least six different women—over the next year—to take Millie's place. None of them lasted longer than six weeks. They couldn't tolerate the routine, or the customers.

About six months before I left Gainesville, I'm doing my laundry one morning. The place is empty, except for me. I'm sitting in the back, reading a magazine and minding my own business. In walks a well-built male college student. Obviously, he's either going or coming from a workout at the fitness center across the street. He fumbles at some of the machines up front, looks around the place, spots me, and walks to the back impatiently.

"Do you work here?" he asked.

Usually, I would have given him a fast, comical answer. But because this was still Millie's place in my mind, I smiled, looked up at the young man, and said: "Yes, can I help you with something?"

"Do you have change for a dollar?" he asked. "The machine up front seems to be out of order."

Since I had four quarters in my pocket, I replied, "Sure," and handed him the quarters. Millie always said it was important to have plenty of extra quarters handy—just in case the machine jammed.

The guy quickly walked up to the front, threw his sack of clothes into the first washing machine, and cranked it up. I returned to my magazine.

"Hey, man," he hollered several minutes later. "I'm going across the street to work out. When the machine stops, could you move my wet clothes from this washer to that dryer?" He pointed as he talked.

Not even waiting for my answer, he hurried out.

Gee, I thought to myself: *What a schmuck. How did Millie tolerate all these types (and worse) for half her life?*

She would have dealt with it, I realized, with a smile on her face—and a helping hand.

So, that's what I did. I transferred that guy's wet clothes to the dryer. I waited around another 15 minutes after my laundry was finished, took the guy's clothes out of the dryer, quick folded them (he had six tee shirts), and put them back into his sack. As I walked home, I felt misunderstood and uplifted at the same time.

That's not the end of the story, however.

"Excuse Me, Schmuck!"

A week later, I'm at the fitness center putting one of my research subjects through a high-intensity workout. The subject happens to be an attractive woman who I'm planning to feature in my *Body Defining* book.

Since Gainesville Health & Fitness contains more than a dozen lines of strength training machines, I usually exercise my people in an upstairs, out-of-the-way area to get away from the crowds and the noise. No one bothers us in this remote part of the gym. But today I'm incorporating negative chins into this woman's routine, and the multi-exercise machine that I use for chins is located downstairs, in the middle of all the action.

So, downstairs we go into the chaos. As I suspect, someone is already using the multi-exercise machine. This guy's doing sets of fast calf raises. There we stand: me with my pencil and clipboard and her with a body that would stop traffic on a busy street. A minute goes by. Then two minutes. This guy just keeps doing more sets. *What an airhead he is,* I think to myself.

Finally, I decided to say something to him. "Excuse me, could we work in for a brief set?"

He steps aside, turns around, and, yep, this calf-raise airhead is the same schmuck from the laundromat. We make only brief eye contact. I'm not sure if he recognizes me or not.

It doesn't matter, however. My trainee is already into position for her negative chins, and we continue with her workout.

Then, another two weeks go by and something else happens.

A Book to the Rescue

I'm good friends with Joe Cirulli, the owner of the Gainesville Health & Fitness. He's in charge of training all the instructors, who number more than 100. Most of the instructors are college students who work 20 hours a week. Every three months, there's an orientation session for individuals who are interested in becoming instructors. Since I wrote *The Nautilus Book*, which is used at the fitness center as a training manual, Joe often asks me to say a few words to the prospective instructors.

Anyway, here I am, dressed for the presentation in a coat and tie, speaking to this group of about fifty young people. As I look out over the audience, seated in the back of the room, is—you guessed it—that schmuck.

After my presentation, there's a 15-minute refreshment break. Several of the people in the audience approach and ask me to autograph their copies of *The Nautilus Book*. As I'm signing the books, several more individuals walk over and start peppering me with questions.

I like such questions because they let you know that, during the presentation, you caused the audience to think a little. As I'm pitching my answers in my Texas drawl, I notice that the schmuck has drifted over within ear's reach.

After several more minutes of chatter, someone asks me about career possibilities in the fitness business.

"Look," I say in response, "qualifying and becoming a part-time instructor at the Gainesville Health & Fitness Center will provide you with a great view of what it takes to be successful in the commercial health club business. But if you fail to qualify [there's an initial written test, as well as a supervised high-intensity workout, that a prospective instructor must pass], then maybe I can get you some equally gratifying work—across the street—at the laundromat."

Because of the way I emphasized "at the laundromat," everyone chuckled, including the schmuck. I still didn't know if he recognized me from the laundromat, but I now had his undivided attention as I moved in for a final jab.

Only Three Things

"After thirty years in the fitness business," I concluded, "there's only three things I really like to do: **train people, write books, and do laundry . . . in no particular order!**"

Again, because of the way I accentuated those last concepts, everyone laughed. Just then, Joe Cirulli asked the group to be seated as the orientation session was about to continue.

Later that day, I had finished training the attractive woman I mentioned earlier, and I was heading out the front door of the club. Suddenly, I feel this tap on my shoulder followed by . . . "Dr. Darden, have you got a minute?" To my surprise, it's Mr. Airhead Schmuck. Except now there's something different about him.

We go out the door together and walk to a more private area. He politely introduces himself to me. Sam is his name.

Yes, he remembers me from the laundromat, and he thanks me for helping him that day. Yes, he thought I worked there. No, he didn't make the connection several weeks ago at the calf-raise machine. He didn't connect all the dots until this morning—from my final comment about those three things that I really like to do.

As a result, we had several good belly laughs—together.

He's not such a schmuck after all, I think to myself, especially since—in addition—he's just asked me several intelligent questions about my book.

In fact, Sam went on to become an instructor—and a darn good one. He even helped me train some of my participants in a later research project.

For the remaining time I spent in Gainesville, sometimes when I'd see Sam at the fitness center, my parting line to him was: **"Do you have change for a dollar?"**

It always brought a smile to both of our faces.

I never helped Sam do his laundry again, but I did advise him how to quickly fold a tee shirt. Sam said he would spread the word . . . not only about quick fold, but also about having extra quarters handy. You never know when you'll need to make change for a dollar, right?

Millie would have been proud of us.

Still Living Longer 33 Stronger

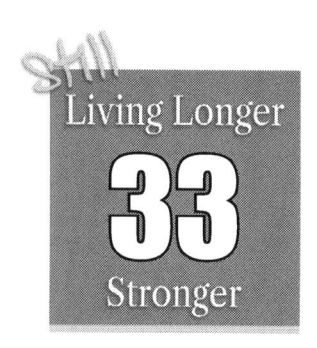

Wanted: Dead or Alive!

Late in the afternoon on December 31, 1995, I phoned Arthur Jones.

"YEAH," he answered in his usual blunt way, which was an indication that his mind was elsewhere.

"Arthur, it's Ell Darden," I said, remembering that he detests small talk, such as . . . How are you? Still, I couldn't resist saying, "Are you doing anything special for New Year's Eve?"

"Matter of fact, I am," he said in a more affable tone. "I'm making a list."

"What kind of list?" I asked.

"A list of the people I'd like to see dead in 1996," Jones replied. "I already have 189 names on it. I'll be finished at 200, which is a nice round number."

Oh my, I sighed to myself, *I wonder if I'm on that list.*

"No," said Jones, reading my mind, "Ell Darden, you are NOT on my list. At least, not yet."

How Arthur produces such shrewd responses, I'll never know. But they certainly are creative and thought-provoking.

Here's another example.

Three Places to Visit

During the summer of 1972, I mentioned to Arthur that I was flying to Munich, Germany, to attend the Olympic Games. Besides being in Munich, I was going to spend another week traveling around Europe.

"Arthur," I asked, "could you tell me your top three places to visit?"

Without hesitation, Arthur said: "I'd rather tell you the places NOT to visit."

Okay, fair enough, I reflected to myself. Negative knowledge is also useful.

"Number 1," Jones declared with an emotionless face, "THE PLANET EARTH."

That brought a short-lived conclusion to a potentially intriguing discourse—which, then, didn't require the mention of his number 2 and number 3 selections.

I always valued Arthur's brevity with words and feelings.

Control, Contrast, and Unexpected

"Arthur's eccentric lifestyle was one of control and contrast," according to Gary Bannister, who owned a Nautilus Club in Caracas, Venezuela, and who spent several weeks hanging with Jones. "One moment he towered over a crowd; the next, he was dwarfed by a horde of exotic creatures (snakes, elephants, crocodiles, rhinos, gorillas), a fleet of commercial airplanes, and a trail of wives."

To Bannister's *control* and *contrast*, I'd add the word *unexpected*. Arthur's behavior was seldom predictable.

An audience of several hundred fitness-minded people experienced Jones's unexpected behavior during a 1983 Nautilus Seminar.

"Why do we get so soon old, and so late smart?" was the way Jones began his presentation. Then, rather than employing his usual lecture voice, he quietly and passionately talked about his father, a small-town physician in Arkansas and Oklahoma who worked long hours during the 1920s and 1930s to support his family as well as numerous relatives.

Jones relived what it was like to grow up in the Oklahoma oil town of Seminole, where roughnecks, gunfighters, prostitutes, gamblers, and thieves seemed to be on every corner. His father treated them all from his home office, with little payment for his efforts.

"In every sense of the word, my father was by far the best man I ever met," Jones continued, "but did I understand and appreciate his efforts at the time?

"Of course not. But I do now, much too late to express my appreciation."

Whatever strength training is, Jones implied, it's not a replacement for family, friends, and acquaintances.

I can't remember the rest of Jones's talk that day. But I can tell you this . . . there were a lot of dads and moms who received sincere calls that night from sons and daughters, telling them how much they were loved!

Wanted: An Influential List

At the start of this New Year, why don't we do a takeoff on Arthur Jones?

No, I don't mean for you to note the people you'd like to see dead in the next year.

Instead, I want you to make a list of men and women (both dead and alive) who've made a major impact on your life.

Take your time and then post—the names, and a brief notation about the *people who have influenced you for the better*. Your parents, grandparents, siblings, a teacher or two, a coach from high school, neighbors, and friends—any or all may be candidates for your recognition.

My List

My dad and mom, George B. Darden and Barbara L. Darden, are no longer living. But I, too, wish I had taken more time, when they were alive, to express my love and appreciation. There are also other men and women who influenced me greatly and deserve my thanks.

- **Hazel Bolin**, 4th grade teacher, who helped me discover the world of books, and, equally important, how to improve my comprehension of what I read.
- **Hazel Briggs**, 8th grade arithmetic teacher, who hammered me with basic math skills and their worth in society.
- **Chuck York**, high-school football coach, who drilled his players with old-school discipline and taught blocking, tackling, and game strategy with simplistic style.
- **Roy Keyes**, high-school chemistry and physics teacher, who progressively made each class challenging and meaningful.
- **Ilanon Moon**, high-school English and Latin teacher, who inspired me to write well by organizing my thoughts in a logical manner.
(Note: The first five people were all from Conroe, Texas.)
- **John Davidson**, professor of theology at Baylor University, who had an easygoing, laid-back style that was full of kindness and wisdom.
- **Ted Powers**, professor of physical education at Baylor, who supplied me with a lot of self-confidence and the ability to "think on my feet."
- **Francis Hall**, professor of motor learning at Florida State University, who shared with me the importance of research-based, precise writing.
- **Robert Stakenus**, professor of educational sociology at FSU, who knew the *why* and *how* of excellent instructional techniques.
- **Harold Schendel**, professor of nutrition at FSU, who taught me the importance of analyzing and understanding the scientific side of food and nutrition.

And finally, much appreciation goes to:

- **Arthur Jones**, founder of Nautilus and MedX Corporations, for his remarkable transition-of-knowledge capacity and for being a master teacher.

Happy NEW YEAR

May this year, and the next, be leaner, stronger, and more productive years for all of us.

Still Living Longer 34 Stronger

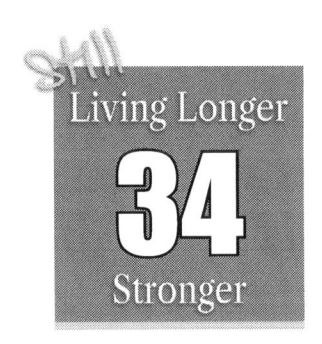

Good Vibrations

Important Notice: This article is a hoax. It is not based on concepts and guidelines that are effective. It is full of lies and misinformation.

BACKGROUND

In 1998, I started a website with the help of Tim Patterson. The name of it was **Classic X**. Classic X was published for three years; then, we changed the name to the New High-Intensity Training.

During the Classic X tenure, I posted approximately fifty articles on exercising and eating. The article that generated the most reader response was the one I'm going to share with you now.

The title was "Good Vibrations: One Waist Problem Solved." The suggested exercises in what you are going to read are not effective. I made the mistake, when it was posted on July 14, 1999, of not telling readers that this was the case . . . until the end of the article in a simple one-line alert. The "Important Notice" tag at the top was not there. Apparently, a lot of readers, and others throughout the Internet who eventually perused it, failed to understand that the article was a joke.

Here's the article.

Father's Day

"What is that?" I asked my daughters, Amy, age 8, and Sarah, 4.

It was about the size of a parking meter—with wrapping paper all over it and a brightly colored ribbon and bow around the top.

"It's your present," they both replied excitedly.

My daughters live with their mother in Daytona Beach and I'm 40 miles away in Celebration. They were visiting me for the weekend. It was early Sunday morning—and it was Father's Day.

I couldn't imagine what this thing was. My daughters arrived the previous day and had been mysteriously working in my garage—putting together that thing—and I had promised not to peek.

So, I carefully tore through the wrapping: first, the bottom—then, the middle. I still didn't know what it was.

"Wait a minute, Daddy," Amy requested as I finished with everything but the top. "Close your eyes. We'll do the rest."

I closed my eyes and stepped away from the thing. About 15 seconds passed as they hurried around.

"Keep your eyes closed, Daddy," Sarah said as she grabbed my hand. "Now step here."

I did as she instructed. I stepped onto a small platform and felt them putting something around my waist.

"Don't open your eyes yet," Amy said. "Just stay there for a minute and see if you can figure out what our gift to you is."

I felt this heavy belt around my waist—then suddenly, it started moving, fast.

I immediately opened my eyes.

What a Surprise

It was a *vibrating belt machine*. One of those devices from the 1950s and 1960s that was promoted to "shake your fat away."

And there I was being vibrated in multiple directions, while my daughters were laughing like a couple of hyenas.

It was one of the most unique presents I'd ever received. They had seen it at a yard sale a couple of weeks earlier—and decided that it would be something that I'd really like. They were right.

The vibrating belt machine was a 40-year-old antique . . . and it was still in good working condition. It was just what I needed to experiment with that hard-to-remove flab around my sides and lower back.

In fact, the rest of the article discusses the reasoning and the routine that I followed to get my waistline to 31 inches. You'll learn the step-by-step way that I successfully applied the vibrating belt machine to shrink the fat cells around my midsection.

Millions of these machines were sold in the United States in the 1950s and '60s. But I seriously doubt that any of the buyers actually knew how to use the apparatus productively.

If you have one of those old vibrating belt machines tucked away in your garage, attic, or basement—find it, clean it up, and get it working. You're going to be very surprised at what you read. And you're going to want to try the two-week routine described.

The Vibration/Fat-Loss Connection

Some of the leanest and most muscular athletes in the sports world are the sprinters in today's championship track and field meets.

Maurice Green, who recently broke the world record in the 100-meter dash, is a prime example. If he worked a while on his chest and upper back, he could place high in a national bodybuilding championship. His waist, legs, and arms are already in superb shape.

What does Maurice do? Sure, he runs—not only on the track, but also in rugged terrain—up and down rocky hills. And he sprints through deep sand and mud.

Green also strength-trains—with heavy weights.

Perhaps most important, after each workout, Green has a vigorous massage.

I'm not talking about something you'd get in the back room of the local YMCA that involves a little kneading and knuckling. Green's masseuse, whose name is Dresden Park, according to an April 31, 1999, copyrighted article in the *Chicago Herald*, hammers him with karate-type chops throughout his muscular system, and especially in his fat-storage spots.

"The deep chops," Park says, "jar and disturb Maurice's fat cells. Afterward, I carefully force the lipid material to ooze out of storage into the bloodstream, where it is eventually removed—probably during Maurice's next vigorous running session."

Interesting, very interesting. Then, Park really drops a bomb toward the end of the story. In fact, what he says is the reason I clipped the article and put it into my fat-loss file. I knew I'd be able to use the information soon.

Park's Amazing Discovery

"Several years ago," Park notes, "I had a chance to buy a half dozen of those old vibrating belt machines from a guy in New Jersey, who had them in storage. They were the heavy-duty kind, which were popular in health spas years ago.

"Out of curiosity, I started using them on the legs of my sprinters. Maurice was one of the first. Others followed his lead. The results were almost immediate. Their bodies became more streamlined. It wasn't long before they were running faster.

"Then I tried the vibrating belts on the men's midsections—and the women's hips and upper thighs. I couldn't believe it. The deep-seated fat started melting away.

"Of course, before I put them onto the belts, they had to undergo ten minutes of my special chopping. Without the chopping, I don't believe the vibrating-belt routine would be nearly as effective."

I tracked down Park several days ago and talked with him on the phone for more than an hour. I told him that my daughters had given me a vibrating belt machine for Father's Day, and that I wanted to explore some self-chopping techniques—with his help, of course—to use in conjunction with the vibrations. My goal was to design a foolproof method for middle-aged men and women to use to shrink selectively those fat cells from their problem areas.

Park was intrigued about pursuing such a project with me. Later in this article, I'll share with you a series of chopping techniques that you can incorporate into your training sessions, which will prove to be almost as effective as having Dresden Park doing the pounding.

But first, I'd like to disclose something Vic Tanny shared with me in 1982. I mentioned Tanny previously in some of my writings. Tanny owned more than 80 successful gyms in the United States during the 1950s and 1960s.

Tanny Talks

"Those vibrating belt machines, or V belts as we called them, were the single most popular piece of equipment that we ever had in our clubs," Tanny said to me one Saturday afternoon at his home on a Daytona Beach golf course.

"You know, we began with two of them in each facility. Soon, we had twelve or more in each club—and the members still complained because they had to wait in lines most days to use one. Finally, we had to put a time limit on them—5 minutes. Some people even started coming in three or four times a day, just to use the V belts longer."

"But Vic," I asked, "did all that shaking really work at getting rid of fat?"

"Only if they reduced their dietary calories at the same time," he replied. "Many did just that, but the credit usually went to the V belt, not the reduction in calories."

"What happened in the late 1960s," I inquired, "that caused the government to outlaw these machines from fitness centers throughout the United States?"

"All the flimsy, home versions of the vibrating belts caused their dismissal," Tanny answered. "I believe a few people actually used them so much that they caused permanent damage to some of their body parts or organs. And then there were a host of other things that many manufacturers claimed helped—like high-blood pressure, arthritis, and acne.

"Finally, the FTC said NO MORE VIBRATING BELT MACHINES. We had 30 days to get them out of our clubs, or we'd be severely fined.

"If I had one today, I'd use it myself. I'd like a little vibration right here and here," Tanny commented as he pointed to his navel area and the sides of his waist.

"Yeah, so would I—or, at least, I'd like to experiment with one," I concluded.

New Sparks

Over the last twenty years, I tried every kind of abdominal exercise and many diets to keep my waist small. Don't get me wrong. I've never had a big waist—ever. It stays between 33 and 33½ inches at my normal year-round body weight of 180 pounds. If I want to get super lean, for whatever reason, I can do so in about a month.

After a month of disciplined eating, my body weight is 172 pounds and my waist measures 31½ inches. But I've noticed over the last ten years that it becomes more difficult for me to reduce those fat cells on the sides of my waist. And they don't seem to shrink quite as much as they used to.

The gift of the vibrating belt machine, combined with what Vic Tanny had told me years ago and my recent conversations with Dresden Park—suddenly had sparked some new ideas in my head.

The Vibrating-Belt Workout

Wow! Something mysterious, indeed, is happening under that vibrating belt. The routine on the machine has already taken 2 inches off my waist, and the fat has evaporated directly from the spots that I needed it most: those side and back oblique areas. Here's the exact routine that I've been using for only two weeks, or six workouts.

- *Straight ahead.* Face the machine. Unhook the right end of the belt, place it around your waist at navel level, and hook it securely in place. Do not lean back yet. Keep the belt loose at first. Turn on the switch. As the vibrating begins, gradually lean away from the belt. Lean away with medium force—not too heavy and not too light—medium. Have a watch with a second hand available. Do 60 seconds of straight-ahead vibrating. Turn the machine off.
- *Backward.* Rotate your body 180 degrees from the machine. Your back is toward it and the belt is over your navel. Turn on the switch. Lean into the vibrating belt. You feel this vibration more in your navel area. Another 60 seconds is called for here. Turn the switch off.
- *Left side.* Turn until your left side is facing away from the front of the machine. The belt should be over your left oblique. Turn on the switch. Do 60 seconds for your left side. Turn the machine off.
- *Right side.* Turn another 180 degrees and place the belt over your right side. Switch the machine on. Try 60 seconds for your right side. Turn the machine off.

That's all for your first vibration machine workout. The following day, check for any bruising. If none is prevalent, your belt pressure is about right. If you notice some bruising, back off on the pressure during your next workout. Repeat the workout on nonconsecutive days, or three times per week.

On your second workout, increase the vibrating time on each of the four movements from 60 seconds to 90 seconds. Preceding each movement, however, perform the following massages and hand chops to the fat-ladened areas:

- *Before straight ahead.* In a standing position, reach back and grasp the skin and fat on your sides slightly above your belt line. You should be holding it mostly between your thumbs and index fingers. Pinch and massage it deeply, back and forth, back and forth, for 30 seconds. You shouldn't squeeze hard enough to cause abrasions, but don't go lightly either. Medium intensity is best. After 30 seconds, go immediately to the straight-ahead-version vibrating movement.
- *Before backward.* Look down at your navel area. First, you're going to hand chop the area where the fat is located. Straighten your hand in a karate-type style. Chop into your middle repeatedly at a 45-degree angle. Do this for 30 seconds. Second, grasp the same fatty area between your thumbs and index fingers and massage it for another 30 seconds. Now do the backward version of the vibrating belt.
- *Before left side.* Hand chop your left oblique area for 30 seconds. Then, massage it for 30 seconds using the same technique as before. Move directly to the left-side vibration.
- *Before right side.* Repeat the same process for your right side that you just finished for your left side.

I practiced the same massage and same chopping time periods for the next four workouts. No added seconds are necessary. According to Dresden Park, 30 seconds of chopping and 30 seconds of massage, if they're done properly, will provide the right amount of "disturbance" to the fatty tissues.

The vibration then takes over.

Park suggests that you progress to a maximum of 3 minutes on each of the four vibration movements. "Three minutes," Park notes, "is about all anybody can stand at one time. You actually become *too fluid* from longer sessions."

During my fifth workout, I accomplished 3 minutes on each of the four movements—and I must tell you—afterward, I felt strange things going on in my midsection. I've done many types of abdominal exercises in my 40 years of training, but I've never experienced this type of agitation.

Good, Good, Good *Vibrations!*

I'm anxious to see what will occur after another two weeks of this routine. I'm not sure if I can get my waist smaller than 31 inches, but I'm going to try. Plus, my body weight is currently 175 pounds, not the almost-too-light 172, which I've experienced in the past when my waist was 31½ inches.

As a result of this new routine, my waist is smaller than it's been in the past, and my body weight is higher.

Good vibrations are happening. I can feel them, and I can hear the music.

Does anybody know Brian Wilson's email address? Let's get the word out to him. I'll keep you posted.

(The article above is a prank.)

Angel Rodriguez

Age 48, Height 5' 8"

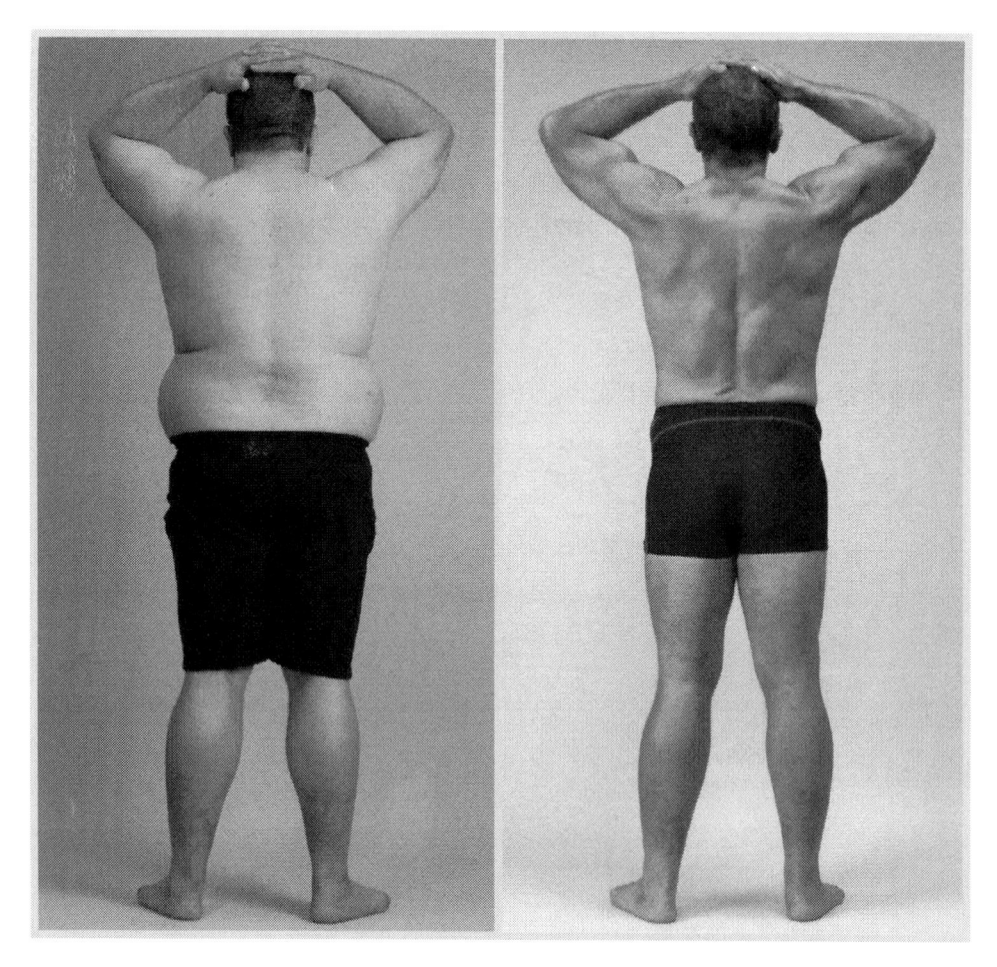

281.5 pounds   **181** pounds

After 30 weeks
121 pounds of fat loss, **20.125** inches off waist
20.5 pounds of muscle gain

Angel Rodriguez did not lose fat by massaging, vibrating, or shaking his flabby areas. Such activities may feel good, but they do not cause fat cells to shrink. The sure way to lose fat efficiently and effectively is through the *Still Living Longer Stronger* program of:

- Negative-accentuated strength training
- Lower calorie eating
- Smaller meals
- Carbohydrates maintained in menus
- Superhydrating
- After-dinner walking
- Extra sleeping and resting.

Angel's fat loss, 121 pounds, and his muscle gain, 20.5 pounds, is the largest fat/muscle makeover (**121 + 20.5 = 141.5 pounds**) that has ever occurred in any of my programs. (See his front photo comparisons in chapter 2.)

You saw in chapter 6 where Boyd Welsch achieved a 60-pound makeover, and so did Melissa Norman in chapter 5. Angel more than doubled their results. And it shows dramatically. Multiple congratulations go to Angel Rodriguez.

Still Living Longer 35 Stronger

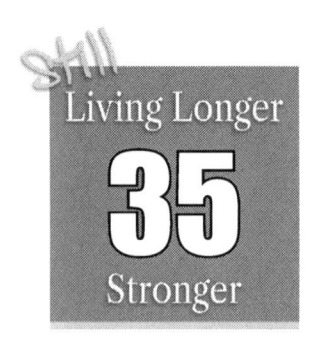

The Rest of Your Life

Worthwhile television. This concept is somewhat of an oxymoron.

There's one television series, however, that I find particularly worthwhile. It's in syndication. The series is *Law & Order*. I never viewed any of these programs when they were originally released, but I've recently watched most of them.

For those of you who are not familiar with *Law & Order*, a bit of background will help set the stage. The location is New York City and, initially, there's a crime that's committed.

The first half of the one-hour show involves two detectives and their boss. They follow the crime trail and usually make an arrest at the end of the first half.

The second half brings the lawyers into the action. Two assistant district attorneys handle the prosecution. In the background towers the older, more experienced, and wiser district attorney. He understands the politics of the city and knows everyone with connections. He doesn't say much, but when he does, it's salient, on-target, and not based on emotion.

The show has been on NBC since 1991. Each new year brought about a change or two in the actors who played the lead characters. But in syndication the shows may not be played in sequence. In fact, they appear to be all mixed up. Monday's program may be from 1995, Tuesday's from 1991, Wednesday's from 1997, and so on.

You can see how this could get confusing. But, after watching for several weeks, it's not—primarily for two reasons:

One, the programs are very well written and produced by Dick Wolf. This man understands television drama. I've not seen a bad episode, and I've watched more than seventy-five of them.

Two, the wise, experienced district attorney has never changed, even though the six main characters have. From the beginning, he's been played by the same actor: Steven Hill. Hill adds that sustaining glue to the entire show. Hill is the show's anchor to reality.

Tennis and Life

Anyway, I recently watched a thought-provoking episode. It involves two 18-year-old girls who were part of the professional tennis tour. They were longtime friends and frequently trained together. One was ranked near the top and was on the verge of being number one. The other was ranked 82nd.

The top-ranked girl has a domineering father who is also her coach. He has pushed the daughter hard to achieve the number-one ranking. As a result, she has almost no social life other than tennis.

The other girl is prettier, and her social life is filled with parties and men. She is also less dedicated to tennis.

The opening sequence shows both girls finishing a practice match and retreating to the dressing room. Minutes after the girls enter the dressing room, there is a loud scream.

The top-ranked tennis player has been attacked by a man, and she sustains a broken wrist. (Sounds like the Tanya Harding/Nancy Kerrigan ice-skating scene from forty years ago, doesn't it?) As a result, her tennis playing is put on hold for at least three months.

Who was behind the crime: A stalker? A lover? The lower-ranked girl?

The domineering father? Or the unexpected?

It was the unexpected. The culprits were both girls.

The higher-ranked girl had burned out on tennis a year earlier. She was sick of her father pushing her so intensely to be number one. She now wanted to lead a normal life.

Thus, the higher-ranked girl, with the lowered-ranked girl's help, hired the lower-ranked girl's boyfriend to bash her arm in the dressing room. With a broken wrist, she figured, she'd be able to ease out of competitive tennis—without embarrassing her father.

The Moral

Here's the back-to-reality lesson from the entire story.

After the plea bargaining and the sentencing (both girls receive probation and 100 hours of community service), the attorneys (the two assistants and older district attorney) are discussing the case as they exit the courthouse.

"It's a shame," remarks one of the assistants in a serious tone, "that the top-ranked girl will not get her chance to be number one."

"Instead," says the other assistant, "she'll be teaching tennis to groups of underprivileged children."

"And she's only 18," replies the first assistant.

Then, Steven Hill, the older district attorney, adds his cogent assessment:

"Most people work a lifetime to get to the top—but this girl got there before her 20th birthday. She ought to consider herself lucky."

There is a pause as the two assistants scratch their heads and ponder that last phrase . . . *consider herself lucky.*

"Now," the experienced voice of reality concludes, "she can get on with the rest of her life!"

True, how true.

Winning, Losing, and Mistakes

Getting to the top or winning . . . when it's happening . . . appears to be "everything," or, as Vince Lombardi said: "THE ONLY THING."

But as most people who've been there realize, such is not the case. Winning and being on top are both fleeting. They are like puddles of water after a rain. They soon evaporate into nothingness.

From that nothingness, however, emerges something that can be of value.

Arthur Jones once said, "Success comes from good judgment. Good judgment comes from experience. Experience comes from bad judgment."

It's not the winning you learn from. It's the losing. You must make mistakes to move forward.

Often, winning reinforces incorrect conclusions. You come away from winning believing you understand the reasons for your victory—which you do not. This sets you up for that eventual fall, which will now be more dramatic because you are in a higher state. If you recover from the loss and win again, then the cycle continues: lose, win, lose, win, lose.

Making Progress

The key to stopping this cycle is to understand the feelings behind both winning and losing. For example, losing hurts, and as a result, most individuals work harder afterward. Winning brings on elation, which causes most people to slack off on the discipline.

Try to eliminate most of your feelings about winning and losing. Look more objectively, instead, at your specific, skill-by-skill progression. You can always get better—*always!*

The secret to long-term progression is to search diligently for your mistakes, mistakes that occur in both winning and losing. Seek feedback from expert coaches and teachers. Identify your faults. Plan, practice, and chip away at improving each one.

Practice doesn't make perfect unless the practice is performed in the most efficient manner according to individual biomechanics. Strive for perfect practice. And perfect practice requires knowledge in numerous areas.

In the long run, knowledge is king. And the transfer of knowledge from one subject to another makes for diversity, which leads to supreme wisdom.

Great Minds

The March 29, 1999 issue of *TIME* magazine discussed the greatest minds of the twentieth century. At the forefront were such people as Sigmund Freud, Albert Einstein, Edwin Hubble, Jonas Salk, and the Wright brothers.

In the write-up about each great thinker was a reference to other men and women who competed against each one to be the first to solve a complex problem. Often, however, the problem was not solved until the competition turned into cooperation.

Competition is good; cooperation is better. But both applied together, in the right amounts, are even better yet. In the best context, competition and cooperation become self-correcting.

In the middle of one of the biographies was this statement: "Failure hovers uncomfortably close to greatness."

Yes, it does.

A hundred years from now, wouldn't it be nice if you're remembered more for your successes than your failures?

A Broad Base

You can be . . . if you broaden your base of knowledge.

When was the last time you visited your local library? Reading stimulates the mind, and the books at the library are virtually free.

Do you have a library card? If not, get one today. And while you're there, browse for at least an hour.

Check out an armload of books. For starters, you may want to peruse some of my favorite authors and their best books:

Robert Fulghum

All I Really Need to Know I Learned in Kindergarten
Uh-Oh
Maybe (Maybe Not)

Carl Sagan

Cosmos
The Demon-Haunted World: Science As a Candle in the Dark
Pale Blue Dot

Harry Crews

Body
The Gypsy's Curse
Classic Crews

Tom Peters

Thriving on Chaos
The Pursuit of Wow!
The Circle of Innovation

Arthur Jones, at more than 78 years of age, used to read at least one book a day. Couldn't you squeeze in one or two a week?

You already know that strength training—*proper* strength training—is the best way to develop your body.

Likewise, reading—reading the *right* literature—is the best way to develop your mind.

Together, reading and training yield awesome strength and extraordinary power.

We're Truly Lucky

Remember what the wise district attorney from *Law & Order* said about being lucky?

Today . . . aren't we all *lucky*?

We're lucky that we live where we have access to competition and cooperation, the Internet, wonderful libraries, quality strength training equipment, and plentiful food.

You've got everything you need to be, and stay, *in control*.

> Now, get on with the rest of your life!

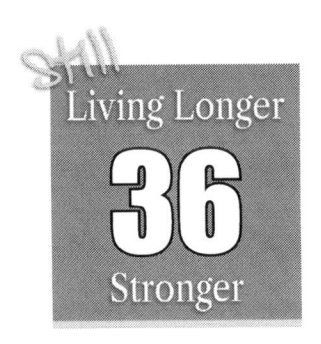

The Transition of Knowledge

Arthur Jones, a master of many endeavors, is fond of saying that much of an individual's wisdom comes from the ability to link knowledge of one subject to knowledge of another. A person who transfers knowledge efficiently and applies it effectively is indeed wise.

John Gray used a similar concept when he wrote his best-selling book *Men Are From Mars, Women Are From Venus*. Better knowledge of each other from both partners' points of view leads to understanding, transition, and meaningful action. The result, according to Gray, is a more productive relationship.

Men traditionally have been more interested in strength training than have women. Yet, it's predominantly women who respond to advertising that touts quick and easy ways to change the shape of the body. These quick-and-easy schemes rarely involve strength training, which just happens to be the best way to reshape. What a shame that so many women are unaware of the effectiveness of strength training and how to apply it correctly in their lifestyles.

On the other hand, women have a much keener awareness of home décor than do men. Yet, most men have the capacity to understand home décor much better than most women give them credit for.

Why does strength training have to be a male activity any more than home decorating has to be almost exclusively for females? A man or a woman, if motivated properly, should be able to master either endeavor.

One key for improved mastery deals with the transition of knowledge. To follow with this thought, I'd like to describe some recent experiences that enlightened me about my body and my home.

A New Home

In December 1997, I purchased a home in Celebration, Florida. Celebration is the new model community of the Walt Disney Company and is located three miles from Disney World. Celebration is designed with a traditional small-town atmosphere, but with modern conveniences such as free Internet access. Most of the homes are within walking distance of downtown, and sidewalks and bike paths connect all points.

The houses in Celebration draw on regional prototypes: Victorian, Classical, Colonial Revival, Coastal, Mediterranean, and French. I bought an Arabella Classical styled home, which is patterned after a design made popular in Charleston, South Carolina, in the early 1900s. Little did I comprehend at that time that I would be responsible for the interior design of the home. I assumed that someone else would make such arrangements. Since I've been divorced for nine years, I soon realized that I'd better do some research in interior design.

I must have studied two dozen books on the subject. After six weeks, I had a pretty good idea about what I wanted. I was partial to a certain southern look: openness, white mixed with greens and blues, and casualness throughout. Since I've learned to travel lightly over the years, I've accumulated only a few pieces of furniture. I estimated that I'd have to buy approximately 75 percent of new furnishings for my home.

The questions I needed answers for were as follows: What do I buy, and in which order? What about quality, delivery times, and cost? How do I blend the big purchases with the accessories to accomplish my desired look? And perhaps most importantly, where do I start?

Two Women With Patience

Fortunately for me, a friend introduced me to Leslie Fogel and Jeanenne Schindele, who are lead interior designers for quality homebuilders in Florida. Both women were willing to do a trade: they would assist me with my home if I would help them get their bodies in shape. It sounded like a great deal, so we all agreed on the preliminaries.

Thank goodness for Leslie and Jeanenne. Besides being skilled decorators, they both have patience. Initially I was completely unfamiliar with the fundamentals they were trying to get me to understand. Then, two events occurred.

To Switzerland and Back

First, I flew to Zurich, Switzerland, to speak to a group of fitness-minded people on my concept of *Living Longer Stronger*. While in this European country, I observed the people. Most of them were obese (like Americans), with sedentary lifestyles, and their smoking rates were on the increase (which is bad sign). Plus, there were few low-fat, low-calorie foods available in Switzerland. The foods were traditional (high in fat and sugar), and the alcohol consumption per person was much higher than in the United States.

Yet, here's the amazing statistic. The Swiss people are at the top of the rankings in life expectancy. Both the Swiss women and men live significantly longer than their American counterparts. But why?

When I returned to my home in Celebration, I was telling a neighbor—Michael McDonough—about my observations in Switzerland. A gifted architect, Michael has resided in Celebration six months longer than I have. Michael's reply started me thinking in an interesting direction.

"The key to the long life of the Swiss people," Michael said, "may be their surroundings. The snow-capped mountains, the free-flowing streams, the rugged valleys, the tall trees—combined with their colorful homes—make a positive impact on their longevity. You know,

Ellington, beauty is healing. And there's nowhere on earth more beautiful than Switzerland."

Beauty is healing.

Could Michael be right in his reasoning? This idea certainly merited consideration.

Self-Extension

Second, a day later, I'm driving my car to the supermarket. On the radio, I hear Dr. James Dobson of Focus on the Family explaining about the primary difference between how a man and a woman view their home. "A typical man," said Dr. Dobson, "looks at his home as being a place he can kick off his shoes, stretch out in his favorite chair, and watch a little TV or simply relax. A woman, in contrast, views her home as an extension of her entire self."

In other words, according to Dobson, a man sees a home as a practical place to get comfortable. To a woman, her home is HER—from the front porch, through the entire house, to the barbecue pit out back—every blade of grass, piece of furniture, and tiny accessory is a vital part of HER.

We can't relocate our homes to a beautiful valley in Switzerland. We can, however, start adding beautiful things to our current surroundings.

I was beginning to make some connections. Your home should be an extension of who you are—and it doesn't matter if you're a woman or a man. Besides being an avenue to relax, it should be a place to revive and rejuvenate. To do that efficiently, it must be appealing, attractive, and beautiful.

Finally, I began to appreciate what Leslie and Jeanenne had been hammering me with for many weeks. They never used the words "make your home an extension of yourself," but they had implied the concept multiple times in their conversations and actions.

Making Transitions

Strength training and bodybuilding are an important part of my lifestyle. I began to apply bodybuilding principles in thinking about my home. For example, symmetry is important in bodybuilding. Likewise, a home should be balanced—at least, most of it should be. But there's a place for the unexpected, such as a piece of art that's different or a room that breaks the mold. You know, like an occasional workout that is vastly different from what you're used to. Then, there's the principle of progression. A properly decorated home should progressively lead you from one area to another, with a subtle theme involved in the background. Sounds like a well-planned bodybuilding routine, doesn't it?

A month later, in June of 1998, I was watching ABC Television's *100 Best American Films of All Time*. During this three-hour presentation, many famous actors, producers, directors, and critics were interviewed concerning their favorite films. The adjective these people used most often, it seemed, was *beautiful*. For example, there was the *beautiful* lighting used in *The Godfather* (1972), the *beautiful* scenery displayed in *Lawrence of Arabia* (1962) and *Doctor Zhivago* (1965), the *beautiful* dancing in *Singin' in the Rain* (1952) and *West Side Story* (1961), the *beautiful* set design in *The Wizard of Oz* (1939) and *An American in Paris* (1951), and the *beautiful* Elizabeth Taylor in *A Place in the Sun* (1951).

Elizabeth Taylor at age 17, according to the interviewed director, was simply "breathtaking." Her 1951 costar, Montgomery Clift, displayed the behavior of a lovestruck man. The look on his face the first time he saw Liz was captured on camera to a degree that could not have been acted or planned, according to the director. Montgomery was swept away by the beauty of this teenage goddess. And it was well known in Hollywood that Clift was gay. Such is the impact of beauty.

Men who have been in the presence of an extremely beautiful woman know what I'm talking about. The instant attraction is inspiring, motivating, and healing—all at the same time.

Enlightenment

Now, I understand.

A beautiful woman. A handsome man. A great build. A lean midsection. Strong, rippling muscles. A symmetrical, buffed body. They are all captivating. They all carry with them a degree of healing and rejuvenation.

There's the natural extension of this concept into the home. Inside, there's a similar feeling of strength and leanness, of sharpness and curves, of squares and circles, of color and lack of color, of the expected and the unexpected, of what's pleasing and what's not pleasing.

People and homes have a lot in common, or at least they should.

I've learned a great deal over the last year about myself and my home: what I like and dislike about colors, casualness, carpet, tile, furniture, walls, artwork, and all kinds of accessories (the little things that can make a big contribution). Although my home decorating is not yet complete, and it probably never will be, I have a plan that is working well. In several months, the initial process should be finished.

My new home is beautiful, and it will improve over time. Having a beautiful home will allow me to better entertain my friends and neighbors and better communicate to them who I am. Since strength training is important in my life, my guests will see the subtle and not-so-subtle connections throughout. I hope my home accentuates the sharing of many related ideas. *Sharing with others* is an important component of my living longer stronger.

The Power of Transition

As a result of my home-decorating experience, I know I'm more sensitive to a person's desire to be more attractive in body, face, hair, and clothes. And I certainly appreciate to a much higher degree the effort that many people put into making their homes more beautiful.

I believe I'm now better able to discuss strength training and other aspects of fitness with both men and women. There's real power in the linking of old and new knowledge.

Take off your shoes and settle back in your most comfortable chair. Before we continue, look around the room you're sitting in. Is there something you can do quickly to make the room more attractive? Yes, I thought so.

If nothing more, you can pick up those magazines on the floor, empty the trash, or straighten that picture on the wall. Do a little something right now.

A beautiful room in a smartly decorated home provides a healing effect. So does a lean, strong body. Your body and your home deserve equal attention.

Apply the *power of transition,* and your wisdom, along with your well-being, will grow richer.

An Update, a Setback, a Game-Winner

My primary interior designer, Jeanenne Schindele, and I became best friends. A year later, in 2000, we were married. We moved out of Celebration and built our new home ten miles down the road in Windermere.

In 2023 we have a beautiful home with all the trimmings—which includes a strength training gym, a swimming pool, three cats, a dog, and two children: Tyler, age 21, and Larah, age 17.

But I digress to Jeanenne's health in 2011.

After two pregnancies and child birthing in her 40s, which was relatively easy for Jeanenne, we had a setback. Her doctor discovered that she had mitral valve leakage in her heart, and she needed open-heart surgery immediately to repair it. Two weeks afterward, she suffered a blood clot and endured another surgery. Then she started a medication that caused her to gain weight.

For six months, Jeanenne experienced a downward spiral in her physical and mental health and put on 40 pounds.

But she rallied.

She helped me rework and reorganize my decade-old Living Longer Stronger program. It didn't have "Still" added to the title yet. She was the first person to jump in with both feet and try it.

During the first two weeks, Jeanenne lost 10 pounds. Those quick results gave her the confidence and resolve to stay the course and transform her body. Thanks to her determined work ethic, she prevailed triumphantly.

Her composite close-ups on the next page reveal the remarkable changes that she recorded over 16 weeks. It was not just about losing fat and regaining her atrophied muscle. It was about taking back the freedom and self-confidence she once had.

Thank you, Jeanenne, for your transition of knowledge among multiple disciplines. You hit a grand-slam home run that won the game. Your wisdom overflows.

Indeed, there's power in transition.

In closing, I want Jeanenne to finish her story.

"It Worked for Me, It Will Work for You"

"Yup, that's my *before* picture on the left of the next page and my *after* picture on the right. I lost almost 43 inches off my tummy, hips, and thighs and 40.5 pounds of fat, and built 4 pounds of muscle.

"I can hardly believe that these comparisons are real and that they occurred to me over 16 weeks. But they are 100 percent genuine. My body change from black-and-white to color in the comparisons was Ell's idea, along with the blue headline and numbers for extra emphasis. He likes them that way.

"Honestly, even if you need to lose 40, 50, 60 pounds or more, I believe this plan can work for you. *It won't be easy,* I can guarantee that. But you'll have Ell's help every step of the way. Mine, too, if you need it.

"You're going to lose fat, build muscle, and then hit a home run. You've got the knowledge and the transitional powers to do them all."

"I was the first person to try the Still Living Longer Stronger Program."
Jeanenne Darden

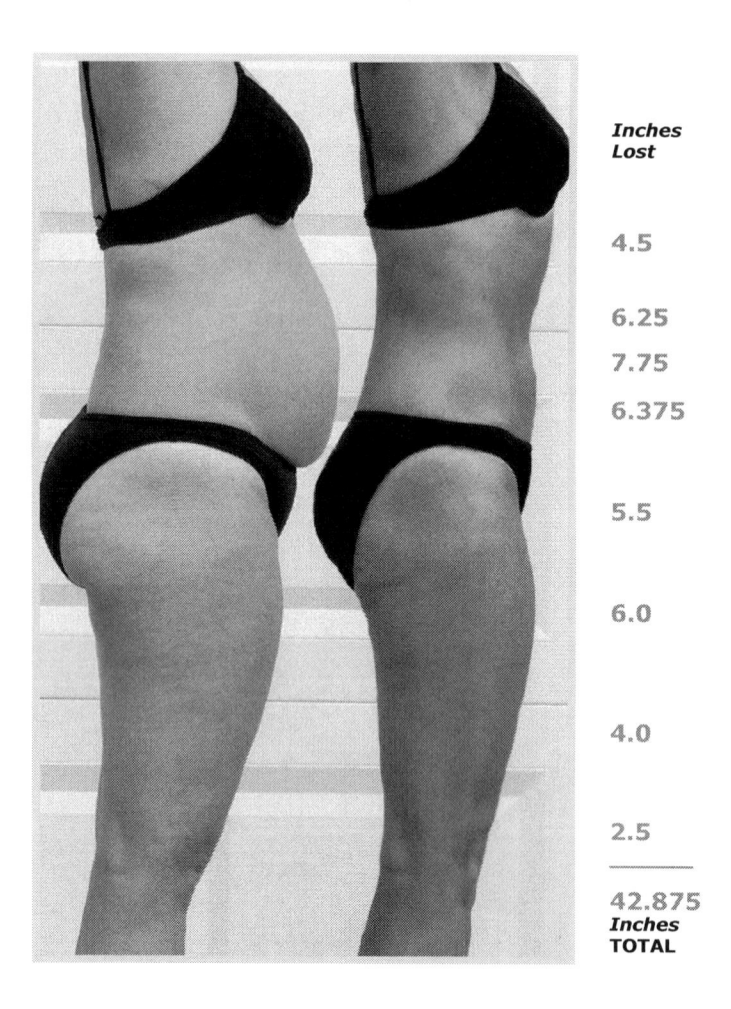

	Inches Lost
	4.5
	6.25
	7.75
	6.375
	5.5
	6.0
	4.0
	2.5
	42.875 Inches TOTAL

A composite close-up of Jeanenne Darden notes her inches lost next to the parallel circumference sites. Applying the SLLS plan for 16 weeks, she shed 42.875 inches and 40.5 pounds of fat.

Muscle Shrinkage & Living Longer Stronger

Between the ages of 20 and 50, the average man or woman loses one-half pound of muscle each year.

At age 50, the rate of muscle loss accelerates.
By 65, inactive adults lose half of their original muscle size. But this is not easily recognized because their fat tissue since age 20 has doubled.

Shrinking muscle is a catalyst for decreased strength, reduced metabolism, persistent dehydration, increased body fat, declining heart-lung endurance, heightened insulin resistance, and continuous loss of bone density.

Rebuilding and building muscle are fast, achievable solutions with the 10-10-10 method of lower-slower strength training.

Muscle controls movement. Muscle rules metabolism.
Muscle powers overall strength. Muscle projects beauty.
Muscle averts falling.

More muscle means more options, more independence, and more success. Your entire physiology can be rejuvenated, and you can live like a 60-year-old until you are 80 and beyond.

Train with Ellington Darden and fast-track your goal of Living Longer Stronger.

Bibliography

Adams, Gregory R. "Invited Review: Autocrine/Paracrine IGF-1 and Skeletal Muscle Adaptation," *Journal of Applied Physiology* 93: 1159-1167, 2002.

Ainesworth, B.E., and others. "Compendium of Physical Activities: An Update of Activity Codes and MET Intensities," *Medicine and Science in Sports and Exercise* 32 (Supplement): S498-S516, 2000.

Asprey, Dave. *Smarter Not Harder*. New York: Harper Wave, 2023.

Astrand, Per-Olof, and others. *Textbook of Work Physiology* (4th Edition). Champaign, IL: Human Kinetics, 2003.

Attia, Peter, with Bill Gifford. *Outlive: The Art & Science of Longevity*. New York: Harmony Books, 2023.

Austin, Daryl. "You Know Protein Builds Muscle, But How Much Should You Eat?" *USA Today*, May 16, 2023.

Bamman, Marcas M., and others. "Mechanical Load Increases Muscle IGF-I and Androgen Receptor mRNA Concentrations in Humans," *American Journal of Physiology, Endocrinology and Metabolism* 280: E383-E390, 2001.

Barrett, Stephen, and Herbert, Victor. *The Vitamin Pushers*. Buffalo, NY: Prometheus Books, 1994.

Beller, Anne Scott. *Fat & Thin: A Natural History of Obesity*. New York: Farrar, Straus and Giroux, 1977.

Berkowitz, Bonnie, and Lindeman, Todd. "Rounding Out the Food Pyramid," *The Washington Post*, June 2, 2011.

Boschmann, Michael, and others. "Water-Induced Thermogenesis," *Journal of Clinical Endocrinology & Metabolism* 88: 6015-6019, 2003.

Bronte, Lydia. *The Longevity Factor*. New York: HarperCollins, 1993.

Bray, George, and others. "Effect of Dietary Protein Content on Weight Gain, Energy Expenditure, and Body Composition During Overeating," *Journal of the American Medical Association* 307: 47-55, 2012.

Brown, S. J., and others. "Indices of Skeletal Muscle Damage and Connective Tissue Breakdown Following Eccentric Muscle Contractions," *European Journal of Applied Physiology* 75: 369-374, 1997.

Butterfield, Timothy A. "Eccentric Exercise In Vivo: Strain-Induced Muscle Damage and Adaptation in a Stable System," *Exercise Sports Science Review* 28: 51-60, 2010.

Cermak, N.M., and others. "Eccentric Exercise Increases Satellite Cell Content in Type II Muscle Fibers," *Medicine and Science in Sports and Exercise* 45: 230-237, 2013.

Chang-Cook, Althea. "Our Favorite Frozen Meals," *Consumer Reports:* 68-75, May/June, 2023.

Cohen, Benyamin. "Einstein and a Theory of Disinformation," *The New York Times*, June 4, 2023.

Coleman, Carver J., and others. "Dose-Response Association of Aerobic and Muscle-Strengthening Physical Activity with Mortality: A National Cohort Study of 416,420 US Adults," *British Journal of Sports Medicine* 56: 1218-1223, 2022.

Colliander, E. B., and Tesch, P. A. "Effect of Concentric and Eccentric Muscle Action in Resistance Training," *Acta Physiologica Scandinavica* 140: 31-39, 1990.

Colvin, Robert H., and Olson, Susan C. *Keeping It Off: Winning at Weight Loss.* New York: Simon & Schuster, 1985.

Darden, Ellington. *The New High-Intensity Training*. New York: Rodale, 2004.

Darden, Ellington. *A Flat Stomach ASAP*. New York: Pocket Books, 1998.

Darden, Ellington. *Living Longer Stronger*. New York: Perigee, 1995.

Darden, Ellington. *The Nautilus Diet*. Boston: Little, Brown and Company, 1987.

Darden, Ellington. *The Nautilus Bodybuilding Book*. Chicago: Contemporary Books, 1982.

Davis, J. Mark, and others. "Weight Control and Calorie Expenditure: Thermogenesis Effects of Pre-Prandial Exercise," *Addictive Behaviors* 14:347-351, 1989.

Edlund, Matthew. *The Power of Sleep*. New York: Harper One, 2010.

Egan, Sophie. "10 Nutrition Myths Experts Wish Would Die," *The New York Times*, January 19, 2023.

Evans, William, and Rosenberg, Irwin, with Thompson, Jacqueline. *Biomarkers: The 10 Determinants of Aging You Can Control*. New York: Simon & Schuster, 1991.

Fairbank, Rachel. "Just 2 Minutes of Walking After a Meal Is Surprisingly Good for You," *The New York Times*, April 4, 2022.

Fairbank, Rachel. "People Who Do Strength Training Live Longer – and Better," *The New York Times*, April 24, 2022, Updated September 30, 2022.

Felsing, Nancy E., and others. "Effect of Low and High Intensity Exercise on Circulating Growth Hormone in Men," *Journal of Clinical Endocrinology and Metabolism* 75: 157-162, 1992.

Ferriss, Timothy. *The 4-Hour Body*. New York: Crown Archetype, 2010.

Fiatarone, Maria A., and others. "High-Intensity Strength Training in Nonagenarians," *Journal of the American Medical Association* 263: 3029-3034, 1990.

Forbes, Gilbert B. Human Body Composition: Growth, Aging, Nutrition, and Activity. New York: Springer-Verlag, 1987.

Forbes, Gilbert B. "The Adult Decline in Lean Body Mass," *Human Biology* 48: 161-173, 1976.

Fridén, J. "Changes in Human Skeletal Muscle Induced by Long-Term Eccentric Exercise" *Cell Tissue Research* 236:365-372, 1984.

Goldberg, Alfred L., and others. "Mechanisms of Work-Induced Hypertrophy of Skeletal Muscle," *Medicine and Science in Sports and Exercise* 7: 248-261, 1975.

Grahn, Dennis A., and others. "Work Volume and Strength Training Responses to Resistive Exercise Improve with Periodic Heat Extraction from the Palm," *Journal of Strength and Conditioning Research* 26: 2558-2569, 2012.

Gray, John. *Men Are From Mars, Women Are From Venus*. New York: HarperCollins, 1992.

Hedayatpour, Nosratollah, and others. "Motor Unit Conduction Velocity during Sustained Contraction after Eccentric Exercise," *Medicine & Science in Sports and Exercise* 41: 1927-1933, 2009.

Hibberd, James. "Arnold Schwarzenegger Gets Candid on Career, Failures, Aging: 'My Plan Is to Live Forever,'" *The Hollywood Reporter*, May 16, 2023.

Heller, H. Craig, and Grahn, Dennis A. "Enhancing Thermal Exchange in Humans and Practical Applications," *Disruptive Science and Technology* 1: 1-10, 2012.

Hilliard-Robertson, P. C., and others. "Strength Gains Following Different Combined Concentric and Eccentric Exercise Regimens," *Aviation, Space, and Environmental Medicine* 74: 342-347, 2003.

Hortobagyi, Tibor. "The Positives of Negatives: Clinical Implications of Eccentric Resistance Exercise in Old Adults," *Journal of Gerontology* 58A: 417-418, 2003.

Hortobágyi, T., and others. "Greater Initial Adaptations to Submaximal Muscle Lengthening than Maximal Shortening," *Journal of Applied Physiology* 81: 1677-1682, 1996.

Hyman, Mark. *Young Forever*. New York: Little, Brown Spark, 2023.

Jones, Arthur. "Negative Work as a Factor in Exercise," *Athletic Journal*, April 1975, reprinted in *The Arthur Jones Collection*, Vol. 1: 299-301, compiled by Brian D. Johnston. Sunbury, Ontario: Bodyworx, 2000.

Jones, Arthur. "Negative-Only Strength Training," *Athletic Journal*, September 1975, reprinted in *The Arthur Jones Collection*, Vol. 1: 317-320, compiled by Brian D. Johnston. Sunbury, Ontario: Bodyworx, 2000.

Jones, Arthur. The Lumbar Spine, the Cervical Spine, and the Knee. Ocala, FL: MedX Corporation, 1992.

Jones, Arthur. "Accentuate the Negative," *IronMan*: 32: 30, 31, 56-59, January 1973.

Jones, Arthur. *Nautilus Training Principles: Bulletin No. 1*. DeLand, FL: Nautilus Sports/Medical Industries, 1970.

Komi, P. V., and Buskirk, E. R. "Effect of Eccentric and Concentric Muscle Conditioning on Tension and Electrical Activity in Human Muscle," *Ergonomics* 15: 417-434, 1972.

Kostek, Matthew C., and others. "Gene Expression Responses over 24 Hours to Lengthening and Shortening Contractions in Human Muscle," *Physiology Genomics* 31: 42-52, 2007.

Lindstedt, S. L., and others. "When Active Muscles Lengthen: Properties and Consequences of Eccentric Contractions," *News Physiology Science* 16: 256-261, 2001.

Lopes, Jaqueline S. S., and others. "Effects of Training with Elastic Resistance Versus Conventional Resistance on Muscular Strength: A Systematic Review and Meta-Analysis," *SAGE Open Medicine* 7: February 2019.

Melby, C., and others. "Effect of Acute Resistance Exercise on Postexercise Energy Expenditure and Resting Metabolic Rate," *Journal of Applied Physiology* 75: 1847-1853, 1993.

McClure, Max. "Stanford Researchers' Cooling Glove Better than Steroids – and Helps Solve Physiological Mystery, Too," *Stanford Report*, August 29, 2012.

McGuff, Doug, and Little, John. *Body by Science*. New York: McGraw-Hill, 2009.

Messier, Stephen P., and Dill, Mary E. "Alterations in Strength and Maximal Oxygen Uptake Consequent to Nautilus Circuit Weight Training," *Research Quarterly for Exercise and Sport* 56: 345-351, 1985.

Murphy, Martha W. "Think on Your Feet," *AARP Bulletin*: 20, May 2023.

Norrbrand, L., and others. "Resistance Training Using Eccentric Overload Induces Early Adaptations in Skeletal Muscle Size," *European Journal of Applied Physiology* 102: 271-281, 2008.

Pacetta, Frank. *Don't Fire Them, Fire Them Up*. New York: Simon & Schuster, 1994.

Pedersen, B.K., and Fabbraio, M.A. "Muscle as an Endocrine Organ: Focus on Muscle-Derived Interleukin-6," *Physiological Reviews* 88: 1379-1406, 2008.

Peterson, James A. "Total Conditioning: A Case Study." *Athletic Journal* 56: 40-55, September 1975.

Pollock, M. L., and others. "Measurement of Cardiorespiratory Fitness and Body Composition in the Clinical Setting," *Comprehensive Therapy* 6: 12-27, 1980.

Rodenburg, J., and others. "Changes in Phosphorus Compounds and Water Content in Skeletal Muscle Due to Eccentric Exercise," *European Journal of Applied Physiology* 68: 205-213, 1994.

Reynolds, Gretchen. "Lifting Weights? Your Fat Cells Would Like to Have a Word," *The New York Times*, July 21, 2021, Updated August 12, 2021.

Roig, M., and others. "The Effects of Eccentric Versus Concentric Resistance Training on Muscle Strength and Mass in Healthy Adults: A Systematic Review with Meta-Analyses," *British Journal of Sports Medicine*: 43: 556-568, 2009.

Sacks, Frank, and others. "Comparison of Weight-Loss Diets with Different Compositions of Fat, Protein, and Carbohydrates," *New England Journal of Medicine* 360: 859-873, 2009.

Sagan, Carl. *Broca's Brain: Reflections on the Romance of Science*. New York: Ballantine, 1980.

Seynnes, O. R., and others. "Early Skeletal Muscle Hypertrophy and Architectural Changes in Response to High-Intensity Resistance Training," *Journal of Applied Physiology* 102: 368-373, 2007.

Sisson, Mark, with Brad Kearns. *Two Meals a Day*. New York: Grand Central, 2021.

Sizer, Frances S. and Whitney, Ellie. *Nutrition: Concepts and Controversies* (16th Edition), Boston: Cengage, 2023.

Sonksen, P. H. "Insulin, Growth Hormone and Sport," *Journal of Endocrinology* 170-13-25, 2001.

Stare, Fredrick. *Your Guide to Good Nutrition*. Amherst, NY: Prometheus Books, 1991.

Streever, Bill. *Cold.* New York: Little, Brown, 2009.

Sui, Sophia X., and others. "Musculoskeletal Deficits and Cognitive Impairment: Epidemiological Evidence and Biological Mechanisms," Current Osteoporosis Reports 20: 260-272, 2022.

Vogel, Steven. *Prime Mover: A Natural History of Muscle*. New York: W. W. Norton & Company, 2001.

Westcott, Wayne. *Strength Fitness* (Fourth Edition). Dubuque, IA: Wm. C. Brown Publishers, 1995.

7 KEYS FOR SUCCESS

1. Use 10-10-10 in your strength training.
2. Apply lift & lower-slower on most repetitions.
3. Eat smaller meals more often.
4. Keep carbohydrates in your diet.
5. Try superhydration. It works!
6. Enjoy after-dinner walking.
7. Get more sleep.

"Muscular size and strength are crucial to living longer. As we age, the muscle we cultivate becomes the elixir that sustains our vitality. With continued workouts, we defy time's grasp and embrace life with vigor. *Stay strong*. Live long."

Dr. Ellington Darden

Bonus
FREE GIFT

Thank you for your purchase of
Still Living Longer Stronger!

*As an extra bonus, I want to give you
a FREE GIFT*

6 week
Living
Longer
STRONGER
M E T H O D

I've summarized the 10-10-10 Method workout program, measurements, and meal plan into a downloadable PDF to make it as easy as possible for you to achieve success while working out in your own home or at the gym.

This workout program is the *exact process* I've taken thousands of my clients through to help them *lose fat, build strength, and improve their overall health* so they can Live Longer Stronger.

To download your free gift, please visit:
livingstrongermethod.com/gift